T0282691

Footprints of the Nursing Profession:

CURRENT TRENDS AND
EMERGING ISSUES IN GHANA

Editors

Lydia Aziato

Adzo Kwashie

Kwadwo Ameyaw Korsah

Florence Naab

SCHOOL OF NURSING
COLLEGE OF HEALTH SCIENCES
UNIVERSITY OF GHANA

UNIVERSITY OF GHANA 65TH ANNIVERSARY READER PROJECT

CLINICAL SCIENCES SERIES NO 2

First published in Ghana in 2014 for UNIVERSITY OF GHANA
by Sub-Saharan Publishers
P.O.Box 358
Legon-Accra
Ghana
Email: saharanp@africaonline.com.gh

© University of Ghana, 2013,
P.O.Box LG 25
Legon- Accra
Ghana
Tel: +233-302-500381
website:http://www.ug.edu.gh

ISBN: 978-9988-647-51-3

Editorial Board:
Prof.(Emerita) Mary Esther Dakubu
Prof. Ama de-Graft Aikins
Prof. Kwadwo Ansah Koram
Prof. C. Charles Mate-Kole

Clinical Sciences Series Editor:
Prof. C. Charles Mate-Kole

Copyright Notice
No part of this publication may be reproduced, stored in a retrieval system or
transmitted in any form or by any means electronic, mechanical, photocopying,
recording or otherwise, without the prior written permission of the University of
Ghana or the publishers.
All Rights Reserved.

Contents

Foreword

The University of Ghana is celebrating sixty-five years of its founding this year. In all those years, lecturers and researchers of the university have contributed in quite significant ways to the development of thought and in the analyses of critical issues for Ghanaian and African societies. The celebration of the anniversary provides an appropriate opportunity for a reflection on the contributions that Legon academics have made to the intellectual development of Ghana and Africa. That is the aim of the University of Ghana Readers Project.

In the early years of the University, all the material that was used to teach students came largely from the United Kingdom and other parts of Europe. Most of the thinking in all disciplines was largely Eurocentric. The material that was used to teach students was mainly European, as indeed were many of the academics teaching the students. The norms and standards against which students were assessed were influenced largely by European values. The discussions that took place in seminar and lecture rooms were driven largely by what Africa could learn from Europe.

The 1960s saw a major 'revisionism' in African intellectual development as young African academics began to question received ideas against a backdrop of changing global attitudes in the wake of political independence. Much serious writing was done by African academics as their contribution to the search for new ways of organizing their societies. African intellectuals contributed to global debates in their own right and sometimes developed their own material for engaging with their students and the wider society.

Since the late 1970s universities in the region and their academics have struggled to make their voices heard in national and global debates. Against a new backdrop of economic stagnation and political disarray, many of the ideas for managing their economies and societies have come from outside. These ideas have often come with significant financial backing channelled through international organizations and governments. During the period, African governments saw themselves as having no reason to expect or ask for any intellectual contribution from their own academics. This was very much the case in Ghana.

The story is beginning to change in universities in many African countries. The University of Ghana Readers Project is an attempt to document the different ideas and debates that have influenced various disciplines over many years through collections of short essays and articles. They show the work of Legon academics and their collaborators in various disciplines as they have sought to introduce their research communities and students to new ideas. Our expectation is that this will mark a new beginning of solid engagement between Legon and other academics as they document their thoughts and contributions to the continuing search for new ideas to shape our world.

We gratefully acknowledge a generous grant from the Carnegie Corporation of New York that has made the publication of this series of Readers possible.

Ernest Aryeetey
Vice-Chancellor, University of Ghana
Legon, August 2013

Preface

This reader *'Footprints of the Nursing Profession: Current Trends and Emerging issues in Ghana'* is a compilation of essays that chronicles the changes that the nursing profession has gone through from the onset of nursing education in Ghana to date. In addition, it also highlights various aspects of nursing practice including nursing management and management of some conditions with a global and local orientation. The reader is made up of twelve chapters and most of the chapters are drawn from the research of faculty members of the School of Nursing, University of Ghana.

Nursing education in Ghana is currently at undergraduate and post-graduate levels comparable to international trends in many countries. It offers nurses in Ghana the opportunity to acquire higher education and skills to provide better healthcare to their clients.

The initial chapter of this Reader reviews undergraduate and graduate nursing education programmes in Ghana. It then discusses the workplace challenges faced by graduate nurses and the fact that nurses who not only provide clinical nursing care to their clients (Chapter 2), but they also manage the wards and perform administrative duties, necessitating a role for nurses in planning (Chapter 3) in order to ensure effectiveness and efficiency at unit level. Chapter 4 looks at the implications for nurses of general and post-operative pain management strategies. Chapter 5 discusses the challenges posed by road traffic accidents for nursing care. The following chapter traces the history of the emergence of human immuno-deficiency virus (HIV) infection in Ghana and the experiences of nurses and caregivers.

This Reader explores a range of issues regarding breastfeeding, abortion, and infertility. These are sensitive and important in every society because of the central role of birth and related issues in the human life cycle. Ghana has a national breastfeeding policy and Chapter 7 discusses matters arising in its implementation. Chapter 8 looks at emerging concerns and strategies for managing female infertility. Similarly, Chapter 9 discusses the policy implications of the effort to curb unsafe abortion and the concerns of the nursing profession and of other stakeholders.

Chapters 10 and 11 explore the management from the nursing perspective of two major non-communicable diseases, namely diabetes mellitus and stroke (or cardiovascular accident). The concluding chapter stresses the need for nurses to conduct rigorous research to develop nursing knowledge and to disseminate their findings through publication in peer-reviewed journals.

This Reader has taken the vast range of nursing issues with the aim of providing an insight into some of the under-appreciated contributions nurses make towards healthcare delivery in Ghana.

About the Contributors

Comfort Afram, MPhil, BA, CMB, FWCN, Lecturer, School of Nursing University of Ghana, Legon.
Research interests: maternal, child health.

Patience Aniteye, PhD, Lecturer and Acting Head Community Health Department, School of Nursing, University of Ghana.
Research interests: reproductive and sexual health, care of the aged, in churches and rural communities.

Patricia Avadu, MPhil, BA, CMB, FWCN, Lecturer at the School of Nursing, University of Ghana, Legon.
Research interest: hypertension.

Lydia Aziato, PhD, MPhil, BA, Lecturer, School of Nursing, Department of Adult Health.
Research interests: surgical nursing, pain management, oncology with special interest in breast cancer.

Ernestina Safoa Donkor, PhD, MSC, BSc. Senior lecturer, Acting Dean School of Nursing, College of Health Sciences, University of Ghana, Legon.
Research interests: women's health and midwifery.

Cecilia Eliason, MPhil, BSc, Assistant lecturer, Department of Adult Health, School of Nursing.
Research interests: care of the aged, and stroke.

Kwadwo Ameyaw Korsah, BA, MPhil, Lecturer, Acting Head, School of Nursing. He is the Acting Head Department of Adult Health, School of Nursing.
Research interests: nursing and communication, coping and chronicity of diseases (diabetes).

Atswei Adzo Kwashie, BSc., MPhil, SRN, Assistant Lecturer, Department of Research, Education and Administration, School of Nursing, University of Ghana.
Research interests: nursing education and research.

Mwini-Nyaledzigbor Prudence Portia, PhD, Lecturer, School of Nursing, University of Ghana.
Research interests: women's health, HIV/AIDS, nursing education.

Florence Naab, PhD, BA, MPhil, Lecturer, Department of Maternal and Child Health, School of Nursing, University of Ghana.
Research interests: psychosocial health problems affecting men and women with infertility in Ghana.

Adelaide Maria Ansah Ofei, Assistant Lecturer, Department of Research, Education and Administration, School of Nursing.
Research interests: health systems management and nursing administration.

Lillian Akorfa Ohene, Assistant Lecturer, Community Health Nursing Department at the School of Nursing, University of Ghana.
Research interests: nursing accidents and trauma.

Chapter One
Nursing Education in Ghana: An Insight into Undergraduate and Graduate Programmes

Ernestina S. Donkor

Introduction

The nursing profession has been sensitive and responsive to the ever changing needs of society throughout the world, and Ghana is no exception. Undergraduate/graduate education in nursing is part of the educational structure of most developed countries and it is intended not only as an academic pursuit but also to help to improve the quality of life of society in general and in particular, its people with ailments. Thus, local specific circumstances determine the needs of such nursing education programmes in addition to universal principles or requirements.

In Ghana, higher education is provided by universities, university colleges, polytechnics and pre-service training institutes (Sedgwick, 2000). Undergraduate and graduate nursing education in Ghana started first in the School of Nursing (SoN), one of the constituent schools of the College of Health Sciences, University of Ghana. Currently, undergraduate nursing programmes are run by both public and private universities. However, to date, SoN is the only school offering graduate nursing programmes in Ghana. As the premier nursing school in the country, the University of Ghana School of Nursing has set the pace for the establishment of undergraduate nursing programmes and has made an immense contribution to healthcare in Ghana. This chapter provides a comprehensive overview of the evolution of University of Ghana School of Nursing and the development of undergraduate and graduate nursing as a whole in this country. Further, it discusses career opportunities, paediatric nursing programmes, distance education for nursing, as well as challenges and future directions.

History

The School was first established as a post-basic nursing institution in 1963 as a World Health Organisation (WHO) Project at the request of the Ministry of Health, Ghana. At its inception, it focused on the preparation of Nurse Tutors to teach in the basic nursing training institutions. Subsequently, a certificate course in Management and a diploma course in Nursing Service Administration were incorporated in July 1970 and 1971 respectively. Thus, at the post-basic level, three categories of nurses were produced (Department of Nursing, University of Ghana, 1990). The diploma programme in nursing was designed to prepare State Registered Nurses for teaching positions in schools of General Nursing, Midwifery, Psychiatry and Public Health or for administration and supervision in Hospitals and Public Health Agencies. Currently, the Diploma in Nurse Education programme is no longer being offered at the University of Ghana; it was terminated in 2000. After 10 years of its existence, WHO's participation in the project was phased out, and the department became a fully-fledged department of the university. The first director of the Post-Basic Nursing Department was Dr. Rae Chittick, (a Canadian); and the first class of diplomates graduated in 1965 (Department of Nursing, University of Ghana, 1990).

In 1980, an undergraduate nursing programme for the award of the Bachelor of Science or Bachelor of Arts degree was started to meet a need for advanced preparation of nurses for leadership roles in nursing education, administration and service. Furthermore, the education of the professional nurse at university level was to develop a liberally educated individual, as well as a professional nurse who would be competent for community health work in assessing, planning and organising comprehensive health services as well as providing primary health care. With the inception of the degree programme, the designation of Post-Basic Nursing Department was formally changed to the Department of Nursing (Department of Nursing, University of Ghana, 1990), with Ghanaian staff led by Ayodele Akiwumi (who later became an Associate Professor). As a department in the University of Ghana, it was administered through the Faculty of Social Studies (now Faculty of Social Science), but belonged to both the Faculties of Science and Social Studies.

The nursing programme was developed to conform to the degree structure of the University of Ghana. Nursing was offered with two other subjects (e.g. nutrition, zoology, botany, psychology, sociology) in both the Faculties of Science and Social Studies. The first batch had two students who graduated in 1984, and the second batch had five students graduating in 1985. Since then, there has been a gradual increase in student population on the degree programme. Currently, about 150 students graduate every year with a Bachelor of Science in Nursing degree.

Since the undergraduate nursing programme started at the University of Ghana, other public and private universities have also started such nursing programmes (Table 1).

Table 1.1   Commencement of undergraduate nursing programmes in Ghana

Institution	Status	Academic year of commencement
University of Ghana, Legon, Accra	Public	1980/1981
Kwame Nkrumah University of Science and Technology, Kumasi	Public	2002/2003
University of Cape Coast, Cape Coast	Public	2006/2007
University of Development Studies, Tamale	Public	2007/2008
Garden City University College, Kumasi	Private	2006/2007
Central University College, Miotso Accra	Private	2007/2008
Valley View University, Accra	Private	2007/2008
Presbyterian University College, Agogo	Private	2007/2008

Graduate Education in Nursing

Graduate education in nursing in Ghana can be considered as the third phase of the university-level nursing education. Prior to the commencement of the graduate nursing programme, the primary mode of providing graduate education was to send candidates outside the country. However, it became difficult to obtain sponsorship for these candidates. Some of those who got sponsorship to study abroad never returned to contribute their quota. This led to an acute shortage of staff at the then Department of Nursing in the University of Ghana. In 1999, for example, the department had only four full-time faculty members with graduate preparation, one faculty member hired on contract and part-time lecturers including doctors / lecturers from the University of Ghana Medical School. While there were vacancies for 16 positions, the University of Ghana was unsuccessful in attracting sufficient qualified faculty for full-time appointment. The establishment of an in-country Master of Philosophy (MPhil) in Nursing programme whose graduates were more likely to be retained in the country (Farr, 2005) was the option adopted to help improve both numerical strength and research capacity of the teaching staff in the university. Also, it allowed the only bachelor degree in nursing programme to produce middle-level nurse-managers and teachers essentially to maintain the quality of nursing services at different levels of the health service in Ghana. In the University of Ghana Strategic Plan 1993-2020, the key goals were to establish graduate programmes in all departments and to increase graduate student enrolment to 30 percent of university enrolment. Approval for the development of a Master of Philosophy (Nursing) programme within the Department of Nursing was granted in 1994, but there were insufficient faculty members to implement the programme.

In 1999, the University of Alberta, Edmonton, partnered with the then Department of Nursing, University of Ghana, to establish a Graduate Nursing Education programme in Ghana (Ogilvie, Opare, Allen & Oware-Gyekye, 2006). It was a five-year project funded by the Canadian International Development Agency (CIDA) as a Tier II project under the auspices of the Association of Universities and Colleges of Canada (AUCC) (Ogilvie, Allen, Laryea & Opare, 2003;

Ogilvie et al., 2006). The focus was to collaborate in curriculum refinement, course development, teaching and thesis supervision for a Master's in nursing programme in Ghana. Further, to strengthen research capacity, and foster opportunities for students. The CIDA project ended in February 2005 (Ogilvie et al., 2006).

The intended purposes of the MPhil programme were to:

- Prepare nurses for faculty positions at the Department of Nursing (now SoN), University of Ghana, to increase the size of the faculty;
- Prepare graduates who can embark on doctoral programmes;
- Meet the need for nurses prepared to assume leadership roles in nursing education, administration and research in the country.

In September 2000, the MPhil (Nursing) programme began with the enrolment of six students. This is a two-year programme that requires one year of course work followed by research and a thesis. Towards the end of the first year, the MPhil students go on six-week educational tour to the University of Alberta to engage in thesis development and build research capacity. They are assigned supervisors whilst in Canada.

Some of the graduates of the MPhil programme have been working as lecturers at the SoN and other universities, and tutors in Nursing and Midwifery Training Colleges in the country. Others occupy leadership positions in the Ministry of Health. To date, 62 candidates have been awarded University of Ghana Master of Philosophy in Nursing degrees. See Figure 1 for MPhil admissions from the 2000/2001 to 2012/2013 academic year.

Figure 1.1: MPhil in Nursing Admissions from 2000/2001 to 2012/2013 Academic Year

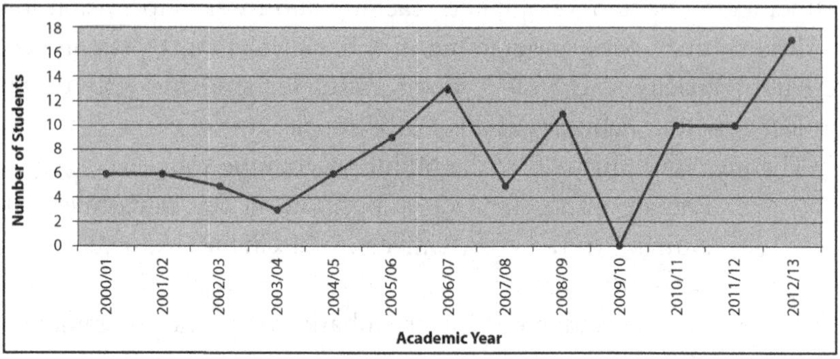

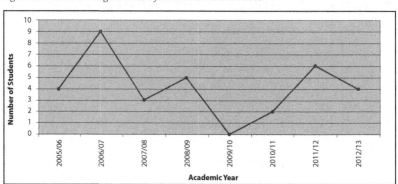

Source: From records of the School of Nursing, University of Ghana

In the 2005/2006 academic year, a 12 calendar month (or maximum of three semesters) MSc Nursing programme was introduced. This was developed to provide an avenue for practising nurses who were interested in sharpening their skills and enhancing their status in their respective areas of practice as bedside nurses, administrators, nurse educators, and community-based project managers. In addition; it was also to provide the Ministry of Health, the largest employer of nurses in the country, with the needed human resource for leadership in nursing administration and nursing practice. The MSc programme requires course work and a dissertation. Applicants must have been practising nurses for not less than three years. To date, 23 students have received the University of Ghana MSc in Nursing degree.

Figure 1.2: MSc in Nursing admissions from 2005/06 to 2012/2013

Source: From records of the School of Nursing, University of Ghana

From a Department to a School of Nursing

From 1999, the Department of Nursing was recognised by the University of Ghana as part of the College of Health Sciences and was consequently operating as a *de-facto* School. It had representation on the boards and committees of the College and participated in the College's activities including the College's congregations.

Early 2003, the then Department of Nursing submitted a proposal to the Academic Board of the University to be considered as a School. The University Council at its meeting on 15th July, 2003 granted the Department of Nursing the formal status of a School in the College of Health Sciences (CHS) of the University of Ghana. The College of Health Sciences currently consists of six constituent schools and an institute, namely: the University of Ghana Medical School, University of Ghana Dental School, School of Nursing, School of Pharmacy, School of Public Health, School of Allied Health Sciences and Noguchi Memorial Institute for Medical Research. The coming together of these health-related schools/institute to work towards achieving a common purpose provides many and varying opportunities. These benefits include collaborative harnessing of the potential of each school/ institute thereby enhancing the growth for each constituent of the CHS. Plans are far advanced for students to take classes together in the courses that are common to the constituent schools. This would foster a sense of networking among the various professionals and provide a common knowledge base and good working relationship for the professional market.

As a School, SoN has five departments, namely: Mental Health Nursing, Maternal and Child Health Nursing, Adult Health Nursing, Community Health Nursing, and Research, Education and Adminis-tration. It is the aim of the School to have all its departments develop their respective specialty areas for students to graduate in them. The Department of Adult Health is yet to develop specialisation in geriatric nursing, cardiovascular nursing, palliative care and oncology nursing, among others.

In the 2010/2011 academic year, when the University of Ghana commenced a four-year degree programme where Level 100 would count toward graduation, the SoN took the opportunity to improve upon its courses. The aim was to enable students to graduate in BSc Nursing with one of the following options: General Nursing, Paediatric Nursing, Midwifery, Community Health Nursing and Mental Health Nursing. Right from Level 100 to Level 300, all the students undertake the same courses. At Level 400, they take the options to give them more focus. In Ghana at the basic level, nurses do midwifery, mental health, general nursing and obtain a diploma in them. Consequently, a nurse with a diploma in mental health nursing for example, will benefit from the BSc Nursing with mental health option. This in effect will help nurses stay with the area of nursing/midwifery that they began with. Currently, this new programme was in its third year of operation.

Affiliation of Public and Private Nursing Training Colleges

The public basic nursing training colleges in Ghana have become diploma-awarding institutions under the Regional College of Applied Arts, Science and Technology system (RECAAST) (Girdwood, 1999). Consequently, these colleges have become affiliated to the University of Ghana under the SoN for the university to award the diploma. A Memorandum of Understanding (MOU) was signed between the University of Ghana and the Ministry of Health on 16 July 2007. The MOU covered three years of affiliation to the university in the first instance. The SoN organised a 'top-up' (to address any gap in content of courses) programme for nurses who completed nursing training college between 2001 and 2007, covering Diploma 1 to Diploma 7 (D1 to D7). The first top-up took place in 2007 and the second, in 2008 for a total of 500 and 1,000 nurses respectively. The third top-up was held from December 2008 to January 2009, and the fourth in June 2009 for 980 and 1,429 nurses respectively. In total, 3,799 nurses were awarded with the University of Ghana Diploma through the top-up programme. The aim of SoN was to cover all nurses who were trained under the diploma programme prior to the implementation of the curriculum approved by the SoN and the University of Ghana. The top-up courses were followed by an examination. A diploma holder who attained a minimum cumulative grade point average (CGPA) of 3.25 was eligible for admission to Level 300 in the BSc Nursing Programme at SoN. (The CGPA consisted of two-thirds based on the grades achieved at the Nursing Training Colleges and a third of it based on examination score attained from the top-up programme). After clearing the backlog for nurses to receive the University of Ghana Diploma through the top-up programme, those nurses who went through the approved curriculum did not need a top-up programme but were eligible to receive the Diploma once the affiliation was in force. Since 2010, with the introduction of the four-year degree programme where Level 100 would count towards graduation, the policy of the University of Ghana has changed and diploma holders are now being admitted into Level 200 instead of the previously Level 300 entry.

It is worth mentioning that there are other private nursing training schools and universities which have established affiliation with the University of Ghana under the SoN for the Diploma in General Nursing or BSc in Nursing for their students. Some of these affiliate private institutions are Narh-Bita College, Nightingale School of Nursing, Western Hills School of Nursing and Presbyterian University College.

Ghana-SickKids Paediatric Nursing Training Programme

On 26 January 2010, a Ghana-Canada collaboration in a Paediatric Nursing Training Programme was launched and a Memorandum of Understanding (MOU) signed in Accra (CIDA/SickKids International, 2010). The Ghana-SickKids Paediatric Nursing Training Programme is a partnership between key health stakeholders in Ghana and the Hospital for Sick Children (SickKids) in Toronto, Canada. In May 2009, the idea of starting a paediatric nursing programme was developed by Isaac Odame, a Ghanaian paediatrician specialist working with SickKids Hospital in Toronto, Canada. The Ministry of Health (MOH), Ghana had also declared that Ghana needed to produce approximately 1,000-1,500 competent paediatric nurses a year to meet the nursing needs of Ghana's eight million children and their families over the next 10-15 years (CIDA/SickKids International, 2010). The Ghana-SickKids partnership therefore aims at reducing child morbidity and mortality rates in Ghana in the context of the Millennium Development Goal #4.

This project was funded through a four-year (2010-2013) Canadian International Development Agency (CIDA) grant. Since there was no specialisation programme in paediatric nursing in the country, building the educational capacity of the SoN, University of Ghana, was critical in the preparation of specially trained paediatric nurses to provide quality paediatric nursing services. The project further aimed to build paediatric nursing human resource capacity in Ghana to have a measurable impact on child health outcomes.

In Ghana, children continue to die in hospitals and community settings from preventable and treatable illnesses like diarrhoeal diseases, malaria, respiratory infections and neonatal causes of death. The infant mortality rate (IMR) is estimated at 47/1,000 live births in Ghana (Population Reference Bureau, 2012). The IMR reported by the World Bank (2013) for 2008, 2009, 2010 and 2011 were 55, 54, 53 and 52 per 1,000 live births respectively. These suggest that there has been a slight decrease in the IMR. The Paediatric Nursing Training Programme (PNTP) was designed to meet the increasing national health demands for quality child care. The main goal was to develop and provide a specialty paediatric nursing programme that has a clinical and leadership focus. Nurses form the largest health workforce, and empowering them with knowledge and skills in paediatric nursing was deemed appropriate to enable many of them to reach out to many children and also to work in the hinterlands where their services would be needed most.

The programme commenced on 30 May 2011. The first cohort comprised 40 participants drawn from the University of Ghana School of Nursing (6), nurses from the three teaching hospitals in Ghana (20), 37 Military Hospital (3), and 11 nurses from other Ghana Health Service facilities in the Accra Metropolis such as Princess Marie Louise Hospital, Ridge Hospital, La General Hospital and Mamprobi Polyclinic. It was envisaged that this first cohort would form the initial faculty as well as preceptors for the programme which is to run for four years. The second cohort comprised 50 nurses. The University of Ghana Academic Board, prior to approval of the certificate programme, insisted that the programme should be terminated in four years and be incorporated into the Master's programme as a specialty. The SoN has started working to achieve that goal.

This certificate programme is the first of its kind in Ghana. The programme, under a four-year CIDA grant and support from the SickKids Foundation, is in collaboration with the SoN, College of Health Sciences, University of Ghana, Ministry of Health/Ghana Health Service, Nurses and Midwives' Council of Ghana, KorleBu Teaching Hospital and SickKids International, Canada (CIDA/SickKids International, 2010). This is a one-year programme designed such that lectures would be offered during the inter-semester breaks, as well as practical training during the university's regular sessions. The ultimate goal is to produce competent paediatric nurses who provide quality care to children and their parents/guardians. Upon completion of the programme, the graduates received an academic qualification from the University of Ghana and a professional qualification from the Nurses and Midwives' Council (NMC) of Ghana after passing a licensure examination.

Prior to commencement of the programme, several committees were set up to cover topics such as oversight, Ghana-SickKids nursing executives, recruitment, curriculum and publicity among others. Members of these committees were both Ghanaians and Canadians, who worked tirelessly through meetings, teleconferences, videocon-ferences and on-site visits to Ghana to ensure the programme took off successfully. A technical working group, Ghana Performance Measurement Framework Evaluation Committee (CIDA/SickKids International, 2010), comprising individuals from the Ministry of Health (MOH) / Ghana Health Service (GHS), NMC, Korle Bu Teaching Hospital (KBTH) and SoN was inaugurated on December 2012 to work with the project team and the oversight committee towards achieving sustainability of paediatric nursing training in the country. It was the intention of the Paediatric Nursing Training Programme (PNTP) partners that the programme be sustained beyond the initial CIDA grant as it would take time to build paediatric nursing human capacity in Ghana. It is worth mentioning that the SoN in the 2010/2011 academic year incorporated paediatric nursing as one of the options of its BSc nursing programme.

Distance Education in Degree Nursing

In the middle of 2012, the SoN started discussion with the Institute of Continuing and Distance Education (ICDE), University of Ghana, to establish a distance education programme for nurses in the country. A training workshop for the SoN on module development was organised by ICDE and took place at Ho in the Volta Region between 30 July and 2 August 2012. Following the development of the modules, the ICDE would work closely with the SoN on the implementation of distance learning for nurses.

The interest in distance education arose from the fact that during admission into our BSc nursing programme at the University of Ghana, the SoN was unable to admit many nurses as it had a limited quota for various categories of applicants. As a result, some of the nurse applicants found themselves in other programmes which their employer (Ministry of Health) did not grant them study leave to pursue. In a bid to enable a greater number of nurses to upgrade themselves to enhance their practice while they continue to provide nursing services at their workplace, the SoN felt it appropriate to provide a platform and also encourage nurses to embark on a distance education programme to acquire degrees in nursing. The aim was to improve the educational level and professionalism of many nurses without creating any temporary shortage of nurses on the wards and clinics in the country.

Career Opportunities

The undergraduate and graduate programmes provide a broad general foundation which enable graduates to work in a variety of settings in the health sector. Some of the graduate nurses have been employed in the field of clinical nursing; others have been involved in research activities, health education as well as offering tutorship in nursing schools. The majority of the products of the graduate programme are found in the nursing schools in private and public universities, basic nursing training colleges, the GHS and the MOH. Thus, the introduction of the graduate programme has helped in developing the human resources needed for nursing schools in the country. Some are working with non-governmental organisations (NGOs) providing health and social services. Others are carrying out consultancy roles in public and private organisations. There are others who are heading the newly established degree in nursing programmes in the country, in private and public institutions. There are others working as administrators in teaching hospitals.

Challenges Then and Now

Starting the degree nursing programme was initially met with resistance from many stakeholders. Placement of the degree nurses was a problem. The MOH appointed them as temporary staff nurses, which was an appointment designated for nurses who had vacated their posts and had returned for re-engagement (Abdulai, 1990). Similar resistance was also faced by these graduate nurses when they started working on the wards. There were remarks from many health personnel such as "Do we need degree nurses to carry bedpans?" "Degree nurses do not know anything", and "degree nurses are theoretical nurses". It is interesting to note that some of the practicing nurses who previously disdained the degree nurses subsequently, took the degree programme. Indeed, the degree nurses were frustrated (Weekly Spectator, 1989).

Those who entered the degree programme with no nursing background had challenges in integration and acceptance into the nursing profession when they started working. There was a lack of orientation and mentoring for some. For others, the transition from student to qualified nurse was a challenge. The newly qualified degree nurse was met with high expectations from colleague nurses who had no degree qualification. There was an inter-generational gap between the newly qualified nurse and the nurses in the field, and considering the fact that the degree nurse was later placed as a nursing officer, there were sometimes conflicts as the older nurses demanded obedience and questioned the respect of the degree nurses. This could be explained through cultural norms. Due to frustration, some left clinical practice and joined mission health institutions (Abdulai, 1990) and non-governmental organisations (NGOs). With time, some of these problems have died down.

The challenges now, are that there are more applicants wanting admission into the BSc Nursing programme but only limited vacancies exist. The demands to pursue the degree nursing programme has skyrocketed among senior secondary school graduates, and some people are even ready to change careers to be enrolled into the programme. Such a challenge calls for more having distance education in order to train more applicants in degree nursing.

Future of Higher Learning in Nursing

There is the need to focus more on specialization in nursing at the graduate level. The School of Nursing will be sensitive and responsive to the needs of society and structure its courses to address societal needs. There will be stronger collaboration with other stakeholders and affiliate schools. Teaching faculty roles will be enhanced through retraining. Exchange programmes will be encouraged to expose students and faculty to new ideas. A doctoral degree in nursing will be offered in the future after upgrading many of our staff to acquire PhDs.

After Higher Learning in Nursing, What Next?

The graduates will contribute through research to the growth of the body of nursing knowledge nationally and internationally. There will be beneficial effects for our clients (patients) in terms of improved health outcomes.

Conclusion

The BSc and MSc nursing programmes were initiated to meet a need for advanced preparation of nurses for leadership roles in nursing education, administration and service. One of the objectives was to equip nurses with higher education in order to improve the quality of nursing personnel employed in the health care delivery system. The SoN is offering Certificate in Paediatric Nursing, BSc, MSc and MPhil programmes in nursing. The ultimate goal is to offer doctoral programmes to extend the undergraduate and graduate programmes, and increase research capacity in nursing and the overall health sector in Ghana. The aforementioned programmes continue to attract many applicants for admission. The paediatric nursing programme, which is the first of its kind in the sub-region, has been established to equip nurses with the requisite knowledge and skills to provide effective nursing care for children and their families. The aim is to help reduce child morbidity and mortality in the country.

The University of Ghana School of Nursing has contributed to the development of the nursing profession and its practice, including research and education. Its programmes are sensitive to international health standards and graduates can engage in the global practice of nursing subject to meeting local licensing requirements.

References

Abdulai, B. (1990). Degree in nursing – necessity or threat? *Weekly Spectator*, March 31, p.3.

A Concerned Graduate Nurse (1989). Graduate nurses too! *Weekly Spectator*, July 8, p.11.

CIDA/SickKids International (2010). *SickKids Global Child Health Program: 2010/2011 Annual workplan*. Canadian Partnership Branch.

Department of Nursing, University of Ghana (1990). *Brochure*. Accra: School of Communication Studies Press, UG.

Farr, M. (2005). Training dedicated nurse leaders in Ghana. *UniWorld, Association of Universities and Colleges of Canada*, 1-3.

Girdwood, A. (1999). *Tertiary Education Policy in Ghana: An Assessment (1988-1998)*. Washington, DC: World Bank.

Ogilvie, L., Allen, M., Laryea, J. & Opare, M. (2003). Building capacity through a collaborative international nursing project. *Journal of Nursing Scholarship*, 35(2), 113-118.

Ogilvie, L., Opare, M., Allen, M. & Oware-Gyekye, F. (2006). Laying the foundation for nursing research in Ghana. In: *Highlighting the impacts of North-South research collaboration among Canadian and southern higher education partners* (pp.97-106). Ottawa: Association of Universities and Colleges of Canada.

Population Reference Bureau. (2012). *World Population Data Sheet*. USAID.

Sedgwick, R. (2000). Education in Ghana. World Education News & Reviews (eWENR), March/April 13(2). Available at http://www.wes.org/ewenr/00march/pratical.htm. [Accessed on 10 August 2012].

World Bank (2011). Mortality rate, infant (per 1,000 live births). Available at: http://data.worldbank.org/indicator/SP.DYN.IMRT.IN. [Accessed on 20 May 2013].

Chapter Two
The Newly Qualified Graduate Nurse: Workplace Experiences and Challenges from the Ghanaian perspective

Atswei Adzo Kwashie

Introduction

Nursing education has seen many changes over the past few decades. There have been major changes from the Florence Nightingale era where volunteers were trained on the job to nurse the sick, through post-basic specializations and currently, university education for the acquisition of undergraduate and postgraduate degrees. These transitions indicate that nursing has undergone tremendous improvement to meet the changing demands of the healthcare system. Nurses can now be recognized as specialists in the various fields of nursing because they have acquired higher education in those fields.

This interest in higher education has generated considerable discussion because it has contributed to the advances made in the profession. These advances have allowed the nurse to take on challenges which hitherto were reserved for certain categories of health professionals such as doctors and pharmacists. Thus, the nurse is no longer seen as merely playing a subservient role in the healthcare system. In addition, nurses themselves have realized that in order to improve care to their clients, they must acquire more knowledge to enhance their skills and status.

University education places one in a position to be a critical thinker. The university graduate involved in critical thinking engages in an intellectually disciplined process of actively and skilfully conceptualizing, applying, analyzing, synthesizing and evaluating information to arrive at a solution and be able to justify that conclusion. The university prepares graduate nurses to translate theoretical knowledge acquired into practice with minimal effort. Graduate nurses are expected to support their actions with assessments and evaluations based on scientific principles. This does not imply that graduate nurses are masters in their field of work soon after graduation. Instead, they are expected to be critical thinkers who can make comparative judgments from data without constant monitoring and with the least supervision. The present healthcare system requires nurses who can function in an environment that demands innovative problem solving. The graduate nurse is expected to fit into this role. With higher nursing education, the nurse is expected to become fully equipped and in order to perform the various functions and roles required in nursing.

Nursing education in Ghana has progressively advanced from basic nursing education in training schools to higher qualifications which are university-based. The newly qualified graduate nurse plays several roles in the course of nursing practice and often has to contend with challenges in the workplace. Success in the workplace can be achieved by overcoming the challenges. These are discussed in the subsequent paragraphs which explore the experiences of newly qualified graduate nurses globally and in Ghana. We highlight the roles expected of graduate nurses in the healthcare delivery system. We also examine the challenges faced by graduate nurses in the workplace and make suggestions on how to maximize their contribution to healthcare delivery.

The Graduate Nurse

Becoming a new graduate nurse is both a complex and stressful transition. Graduates must settle into the context of nursing practice, become accountable for patient care and ward activities, interact with other health professionals and develop their own clinical expertise (Newton & McKenna, 2007). According to Newton and McKenna (2007), new nursing graduates experience stress and feelings of being unprepared on entering the nursing workforce for the first time. Professional socialization for new graduates involves adjusting to new roles, increasing accountability for patient care, coping with fears of making mistakes or interacting with other health professionals. These graduates move through phases, initially internalizing, focusing on themselves, before being able to work independently and focus on patient and ward requirements.

New graduate nurses are expected to posses the necessary competence to perform their roles and functions as nurses. Regarding their socialization, they either fit in or assume the beliefs and behaviours of their organization, or they can leave, or tolerate rejection (Goh & Watt, 2003). Despite this pressure, graduates did not forfeit their professional values in the work environment, but rather strived to achieve high standards and remain committed to the nursing profession.

Deloughery (1998) gives a list of competencies expected of the graduate nurse in accordance with the National League for Nursing (NLN) in the United States. The NLN (1987) expects the graduate from a university-based programme in nursing is prepared to perform the following:

1. Provide professional nursing care, including health promotion and maintenance, illness care, restoration, rehabilitation, health counselling, and education based on knowledge derived from theory and research;
2. Synthesize theoretical and empirical knowledge from nursing, scientific, and humanistic disciplines with nursing practice;
3. Use the nursing process to provide nursing care for individuals, families, groups and communities;
4. Accept responsibility and accountability for the evaluation of the effectiveness of their nursing practice;
5. Enhance the quality of nursing and health practices within practical settings through the use of leadership skill and a knowledge of the political system;
6. Evaluate research for the applicability of its findings to nursing practice;
7. Participate with other health care providers and members of the public in promoting general health and well-being;
8. Incorporate professional values and ethical, moral, and legal aspects of nursing into nursing practice; and
9. Participate in implementation of nursing roles designed to meet emerging health needs of the general public in a changing society (NLN, 1987, cited in Deloughery, 1998).

These competencies, although set in the context of the US, can be applied to the Ghanaian setting. This is so because graduates from university-based programmes in Ghana perform similar functions in the workplace.

Nurses trained at the School of Nursing, University of Ghana, Legon, go through a four-year programme acquiring education in biomedical sciences and nursing science. There are two categories of graduate nurses in Ghana. The first group comprises registered nurses who have already gone through a nursing programme and have entered the university to acquire education leading to the award of a degree in nursing. The second group is those students who have come straight from secondary school (generics). They all undergo the four-year programme, which leads to the award of the degree in nursing, and then proceed to write a licensure examination which qualifies them to practice as professional nurses.

Irrespective of which mode of entry into the university programme, graduate nurses in Ghana provide services nationwide which can be seen in the form of caregivers, client advocates, change agents, case finders, consultants, teachers and leaders. As caregivers, graduate nurses provide care to client, family or community depending on the setting. It may be in the hospital or home or within the community. In playing the role of an advocate, the graduate nurses become the mouthpiece of the client and act on behalf of the client to ensure well-being. As a change agent, their training and education prepare them to identify situations that need to be changed to ensure the safety and well-being of people. By using their skills in communication, the change needed can be effected. Nurses are almost always engaged in patient teaching and the graduate nurses are not left out of this endeavour. As consultants, graduate nurses can be consulted by their colleagues and clients for advice and possible solutions to some problems. As case finders, the graduate nurses are able to identify clients who need medical attention or otherwise and help them receive the needed attention.

After completing their programme of study, graduate nurses are expected to take up positions in the practical setting and provide nursing care to clients in the health care delivery system. In the course of work, they may decide to pursue further education to acquire postgraduate degrees. The initial nursing experiences of new graduate nurses most often occur in the context of the clinical setting of health service organization. At this point, it is worth noting that newly qualified graduate nurse in this context refers to the one who does not have prior nursing experience before entering the university (generics) to acquire a degree in nursing. These graduate nurses have to provide nursing care alongside the nurses already in the health care delivery system some of whom would be holders of diplomas and auxiliary nurses. By virtue of their education and qualification, they may be placed in a higher position soon after graduation and be working with someone who has several years of experience but no degree. They are faced with many challenges and resentment coming from such colleagues as they have to meet the responsibilities associated with their positions of employment. So much is expected from them, especially from the nurse-managers and also other nurses in the workplace (Kwashie, 2007)

There are differences of opinion about nurses who have graduated from the university with respect to their service provision (which includes clinical practice and patient management). Many nurses with diplomas from the nursing training schools already working but who do not have university degrees have complained that graduate nurses are inadequately prepared for service provision at the time of graduation. The clinical practice hours for the diploma programmes as prescribed by the Nurses and Midwives Council of Ghana is for the students to have fourteen (14) weeks of clinical practice per year for three years before students graduate. At the University, the students have twelve (12) weeks per year for four years after which they graduate.

Experiences of New Graduate Nurses

Various nursing researchers define newly graduated nurses as practitioners who have either graduated from a college of nursing within the last year, or nurses who have practiced for one year or less (Delaney, 2003; Dyess & Sherman, 2009; Oermann & Garvin, 2002). Kramer (1975) used the term neophyte to describe a newly registered nurse who has graduated from an associate, diploma, or baccalaureate programme within the last year or two and transitioned into a medical centre or hospital. The movement from the school setting into nursing practice stirs up a lot of emotion, some of which are helplessness, frustration, powerlessness and dissatisfaction. In addition, the new graduate nurses experience reality shock, an experience found to be a common occurrence in the first stage of role transitioning. This experience comes with moving from the known role of a student to the relatively less familiar role of the professionally practicing nurse (Duchscher, 2009). The experiences come in the form of the relationships, roles, responsibilities, knowledge and performance expectations required within the more familiar academic environment and those required in the professional practice setting.

A study was carried out at Korle Bu Teaching Hospital in Accra, Ghana on the experiences of newly qualified graduate nurses. Findings showed that workplace experiences of graduate nurses include the lack of proper orientation and mentoring to become proficient, difficulty in being accepted as a member of the health team, assuming the responsibility of being a ward manager and displaying the ability to deal with challenges that arise in the course of work. These new graduates complained that the lack of proper orientation and a mentor to assist with becoming proficient affects the new graduate nurse as he/she has to "fit" into the workplace with little or no orientation, no formal job description and limited practical experience. Those who had recently graduated expressed the desire to be part of the unit culture, in that this fosters good interpersonal relationships thereby allowing one to feel a part of a larger group or team which is working to achieve a common goal. One has to work hard to overcome the sometimes negative attitudes and at the same time strive hard to meet expectations of others, irrespective of the fact that one is only newly qualified and is now learning the ropes of the new role (Kwashie, 2007). Many newly graduated nurses have reported experiencing difficult relationships with numerous individuals, including peers, physicians, managers, and preceptors throughout the orientation process and transition period. They felt they were neither respected, nor accepted, by more experienced nurses and other members of the health team.

They expressed frustration with preceptors, or experienced nurses, who no longer showed understanding of newly graduated nurses and their needs (Bowles & Candela, 2005).

Nonetheless, there have been other experiences that served as motivation for the newly qualified graduate nurses. The fact that they have earned their professional licence to practice nursing on graduation is very emotional for them. There are positive feelings of pride and accomplishment knowing that they have become nurses. Some have shared feelings of confidence and excitement to be finally with patients, nursing them and using their skills acquired from school (Dyess & Sherman, 2009).

Challenges Facing New Graduate Nurses

When newly graduated nurses were asked by Fink, Krugman, Casey and Goode (2008) to identify stressors which were present during the first six months of transitioning into healthcare settings, they listed the National Council for Licensure (NCLEX) preparation and results, leaving home or moving out of state, and adjusting to new work environments and professional responsibilities. They developed themes to organize respondents' ideas regarding their transitional period; nearly all of the participants (399, or 92 percent) reported five challenges. These challenges, or five role transition difficulties, were identified as: role changes, workload, orientation issues, fears, and lack of confidence (Fink et al., 2008). Two of the five difficulties, fears and lack of confidence, were centred on new graduates' emotional experiences. The research participants, newly graduated nurses, reported fears of harming patients, making medication errors, losing their license, not providing safe care, and failing to meet colleagues' expectations. In addition to the fears of harming patients, the new graduate registered nurses stated that they lacked confidence in their ability to clearly communicate with physicians and patients, perform skills and assessments, delegate tasks, and think critically.

In Ghana, challenges facing newly qualified graduate nurses are similar to those mentioned above. They include being accepted as a member of the health team, taking up responsibilities as a ward manager, translating theory into practice, managing workload, meeting the expectations of their superiors as well as colleagues and ensuring that the care they provide is adequate and appropriate (Kwashie, 2007).

New graduates also experience challenges with role changes. Role changes such as independent practice, assertiveness, responsibility (registered nurse versus student), preceptor, charge nurse, and personal role were all difficult and challenging. Role changes identified included being prematurely placed in the positions of charge nurse or in the role of preceptor, being asked to delegate tasks to unlicensed assistants with whom they used to work, or being dependent on nursing colleagues when independence was desired (Fink et al., 2008). Struggling to overcome these challenges leads to the adoption of various strategies which these nurses have found useful to enable them stay in the profession and survive in the world of work.

Overcoming the Challenges

Bowles and Candela (2005) found that during the first year of work, also called the transition period, graduate nurses found that by utilizing self-reflection techniques they could evaluate and reframe experiences, understand their place within organizations and the nursing profession, and adapt to workplace environments throughout the transition phase. Delaney (2003) identified this as an important process enabling new graduates to move forward. Intense self-evaluation and personal reflection helped them resolve conflicts and leads to improved self-confidence. Spending time to think about what transpired during one's shift helped to organise and prepare for what might happen on the next shift.

A study on workplace experiences of newly qualified generic graduate nurses by Kwashie (2007) at the KorleBu Teaching Hospital, Accra, identified various ways that new nurse graduates cope with challenges they face at the workplace. Personal coping strategies adopted by a few nurses in this study included being humble, showing respect to already existing nurses on the wards irrespective of their rank and also being punctual to work. They found out that their status as graduate nurses puts pressure on them to perform creditably in all circumstances. However, they were newly qualified and felt that they needed some time to find their feet. Since they came to meet the other nurses on the ward who might not necessarily be graduates but have years of experience on the job, the graduate nurses had to humble themselves and allow these nurses to help them out. One nurse expressed the feeling that it was only a matter of time and the competence for clinical skills would be acquired. Unfortunately, the perception that new graduates possess a low level of clinical competence creates tension among colleagues and employers. What seems to be forgotten is that the novice practitioners need to develop skills in judgment and organization before they can function as effective registered nurses. In this study, the graduate nurses acknowledged this need. In cases where their colleagues on the ward failed to realise this need, the new graduates just 'came down to their level', to learn and within a short time, they were well prepared to take on higher nursing assignments, especially those related to clinical skills.

Punctuality also came out strongly as a personal coping strategy. Punctuality was important for ensuring safe and efficient practice. Adopting the attitude of reporting to work on time facilitated new graduate nurses being easily recognised and accepted as part of the health team. They would then be given the needed support and guidance which in turn boosts their morale and enables them to give off their best at work. Respecting older colleague nurses irrespective of their rank was another coping mechanism cited by a few of the participants in the study by Kwashie (unpublished data). They believed that sometimes working alongside someone older than you but not as educated was a natural thing that may occur at workplaces. The potential for these young graduates to advance faster academically and be offered better conditions of service is a fact which cannot be overlooked. They agreed that it was an advantage for them to have the opportunity to advance academically with their current level of education. However, the generic nurses wanted to work and become proficient and they would need the assistance of the older nurses in all their endeavours. In the Ghanaian cultural context, children are socialised to respect elders at all times even if the younger person may have advanced to a higher level of education than the older person. Sometimes this form of socialisation may be seen in the workplace. Parties in this kind of informal relationship are able to co-exist and allow the work to progress successfully. The respondents who used this approach reported a good working relationship with their colleagues. By showing respect, they were able to do extremely well in the workplace and their work output was very good.

Achieving Success in the Socialization Process

Registered nurse residency programmes offer multiple benefits in the socialization process for the new graduate nurse. Registered nurse residency programmes have become an expectation of newly graduated nurses when seeking employment for their first job. The orientation programmes are to foster integration into the system and nursing profession, encourage creative thinking, and promote skills of lifelong learning. Currently, the practice in Ghana is to have a one-year programme called rotation for such nurses where they are given orientation in specialty areas. By the end of the period, the nurses who go through this process are able to demonstrate improved critical-thinking ability, socialization, stress management, and problem-solving skills. All new employees require orientation at their workplace and newly qualified graduate nurses are no exception.

Mentoring can be applied in nursing the same way as it is done in other professions. This is a non-supervisory role in which an experienced senior colleague provides guidance and encouragement to the fresh graduate at work. This way, the new graduate nurse can build confidence in applying theoretical knowledge to solve problems, formulate appropriate plans of care, implement nursing interventions in a timely manner and evaluate the outcome of intervention. Every registered nurse also enters the profession as an advanced beginner practitioner. Thus, as the novice or advanced beginner moves forward in the journey of clinical experience, the desired outcomes of nursing care are achieved (Hom, 2003). Therefore, during the first two years of clinical practice, the new graduate nurse requires time to solidify skills as well as consistently demonstrate a level of safe and competent care. Since nursing has traditionally been taught more from the practical than theoretical approach, newly qualified graduate nurses tend to feel apprehensive about their ability to be effective in their early days of practice. This is made worse by the reported contemporary tertiary nursing education. Much of this criticism has been levelled either at the gap between theory and practice, or education and service (Pigott, 2001). Like any profession, coming into nursing from a more theoretical and analytical level presents some challenges during the early practice days. With the help of a mentor to encourage and act as a sounding board for new ideas, these challenges easily become opportunities for the graduate nurses to translate their theoretical knowledge into skilful practice.

A formal mentoring programme linking new graduate nurses to seasoned senior nurses would enable them to fit more easily into the workplace, enhance their ability to confidently apply their knowledge and enable them to develop their full potential in the profession. It therefore becomes important that there is a person willing to mentor them in order for these new graduates fit into the work place without much difficulty. Some new graduates accept that they are not adequately prepared for what they are likely to encounter when they are employed in the hospitals. When there is support and guidance, it ensures that safe and efficient practice is maintained and continues to develop. Thus, mentoring new graduate nurses by providing orientation to hospital environments, involving them in decision making, and assisting them to become familiar with different equipment, hospital policies and procedures will reduce the difficulties graduate nurses face in their first year of practice. The newly qualified graduate nurses need support as they are the future leaders of the nursing profession. New graduates have a latent practical ability that can readily be transferred to the clinical setting given an appropriate level of support and guidance through mentorship.

The importance of and need for reflective practice is also relevant to the socialization process for new nurse graduates. Reflection creates self-awareness and its impact on nurses is profound (Schipper, 2011). Being able to take time for newly graduated nurses to articulate and share tales of patient care is essential in developing a well-rounded and balanced nurse who has to deal with various situations and conditions that occur during nursing care of clients. Storytelling and self-reflection are healing for the nurse whose story is being told and allows other newly graduated nurses to share and gain knowledge related to another's experience. Reflection needs to be supported and facilitated by a professional colleague who is able to facilitate the learning that occurred and aid the new nurse in identifying ways to learn from these experiences. Giving newly qualified nurses time to reflect and brainstorm alternative endings to how a particular event occurred contributes to the environment of trust. In asking questions such as "how would you handle that next time?" "what would you do differently?" and "what are you most proud of?" supports, empowers, heals, and nurtures the nurses and provides supportive peer feedback, socialization and strength from the support network (Schipper, 2011). Thus, they are able to translate the new knowledge derived from the reflection into practice and provide better care to their clients. This gives a feeling of satisfaction, confidence and also drives them to excel at work.

Conclusion

During the last few decades, nursing education has been transformed to align with changing healthcare trends, evolving from primarily an apprenticeship-training model to a higher education model. Some countries have standardized the educational preparation for entering registered nurse practice to a baccalaureate degree. As stated earlier, in Ghana, there are two entry levels for registered nurses. These are the university prepared (baccalaureate) and the diploma entry. This paper has focused on the graduate nurse from the university. Concerns about new graduates and their readiness for practice persist in spite of significant advancements in the foundational educational preparation of nurses. The perceived lack of readiness for practice is commonly stated as the rationale for researchers assessing the clinical competence and the performance of beginning practitioners. Research on the perceived lack of new graduates who demonstrate readiness for practice has primarily focused on the transition of students and new graduates into practice. It is important to document the experiences of newly qualified graduate nurses at their workplace. In the Ghanaian context, the fact that there are two entry levels brings out the differences in the competence of diploma and degree nursing graduates. Exploring the experiences and challenges faced by the newly qualified graduate nurse has provided evidence pertinent to the best way to educate nurses to meet the expectations of employers in the healthcare sector. It also offers opportunities for nurse educators to identify whether or not new graduate nurses are ready for registered nurse roles. Collaboration between both faculty and clinicians will enable all stakeholders to work towards ensuring that the nurse graduates are 'practice ready' on graduation and can meet the demands of the healthcare system.

References

Bowles, C., & Candela, L. (2005). First job experiences of recent RN graduates: improving the work environment. *Journal of Nursing Administration*, 35(3), 130–137.

Delaney, C. (2003). Walking a fine line: Graduate nurses' transition experiences during orientation. *The Journal of Nursing Education*, 42(10), 437.

Deloughery, G. L. (1998). *Issues and trends in nursing*. Mosby Inc.

Duchscher, J. E. B. (2009). Transition shock: the initial stage of role adaptation for newly graduated Registered Nurses. *Journal of Advanced Nursing*, 65(5), 1103–1113.

Dyess, S. M., & Sherman, R. O. (2009). The first year of practice: New graduate nurses' transition and learning needs. *The Journal of Continuing Education in Nursing*, 40(9), 403.

Fink, R., Krugman, M., Casey, K., & Goode, C. (2008). The graduate nurse experience: Qualitative residency program outcomes. *Journal of Nursing Administration*, 38(7/8), 341–348.

Goh,K. & Watt, E. (2003). From 'dependent on' to 'depended on': the experience of transition from student to registered nurse in a private hospital graduate program. *Australian Journal of Advanced Nursing*, 21 (1),14-20.

Hom, E. M. (2003). Coaching and mentoring new graduates entering perinatal nursing practice. *The Journal of Perinatal and Neonatal Nursing*, 17(1), 35–49.

Kramer, M. (1975). Reality shock: Why nurses leave nursing. *The American Journal of Nursing*, 75(5), 891.

Kwashie, A. (2007) (Unpublished data).MPhil Thesis. *Workplace Experiences of Newly Qualified Generic Graduate Nurses*. University of Ghana, Legon.

National League for Nursing. (1987). Competencies of the associate degree nurse on entry into practice. In: Deloughery, G. L. (1998). *Issues and Trends in Nursing*. Mosby Inc.

Newton,J.M. & McKenna,L. (2007). The transitional journey through graduate year. A focus group study. *International Journal of Nursing Studies*, 44(7), 1231-1237

Oermann, M. H., & Garvin, M. F. (2002). Stresses and challenges for new graduates in hospitals. *Nurse Education Today*, 22(3), 225.

Pigott, H. (2001). Facing reality: The transition from student to graduate nurse. *Australian Nursing Journal:* 8(7), 24.

Schipper, L. M. (2011). The Socialization Process of Newly Graduated Nurses Into a Clinical Setting: Role of the Clinical Nurse Educator. *Journal for Nurses in Staff Development*, 27(5), 216.

Chapter Three
Planning: The Role of Nurse-Managers at the Unit Level
Adelaide Maria Ansah Ofei

Introduction

Today, clinical health organizations are facing new challenges that have affected a variety of professions, particularly nursing (Danielson & Berntsson, 2007; Mohr et al., 2008; Ford, 2009). These challenges come in the form of new technology that requires new skills, increased workload, shortage of qualified personnel, and decreased resources. Nursing is in a unique position to address challenges that plague the nation's health system. The nurse-manager represents an exciting and promising opportunity for nursing to take a leadership role, in collaboration with multiple practice partners, and implement quality improvement and patient safety initiatives across all healthcare settings. Nurse-managers are responsible for an individual unit or ward (Duffield, 1991) and have a pivotal role in establishing a professional practice environment for delivery of patient care that is conducive to staff satisfaction (Zori, Nosek & Musil, 2010).

The nurse manager, however, will have to plan in order to be efficient and effective. Planning is widely acknowledged as fundamental to organizational life and reaffirms the organization's competitive edge among other players within the industry. The following topics are discussed below: theoretical basis of planning, the planning process, benefits of planning, roles of the nurse-manager, and factors influencing planning.

Background

Nurse-managers play a key role in achieving a healthcare organization's goals of delivering high-quality care to satisfied patients, and creating a positive work environment which fosters staff satisfaction (McGuire & Kennerly, 2006) and financial sustainability. Nurse-managers must have a strategy for accomplishing more with decreasing resources, (Ohman, 2000; Robbins & Davidhizar, 2007) that results in high-quality cost-effective patient care, as well as high levels of patient satisfaction (Casida & Pinto-Zipp, 2008). As a strategy for attaining these goals, the nurse-manager has to plan for taking charge of the day-to-day running of the unit.

Planning has been defined as a process of deciding in advance what to do, how to do it, when to do it, and who should do it (Marquis & Huston, 2006 p, 146). This bridges the gap from where an organization is to where it wants to be. Planning is an important self-regulatory tool that enables efficient progress towards goal attainment and has been proposed as an influential strategy in the translation of intentions into behaviour. Thoughtful planning results in a blueprint, showing the action steps necessary for the achievement of future goals. The planner sets the objectives to be attained and sets a timeline to monitor the progress of the plan (McEachen & Keogh, 2007).

The front-line nurse-manager in Ghana is usually a Senior Nursing Officer who is regarded as either the ward manager or unit-in-charge. The front-line nurse-manager gets to this position through progressive promotions from either a staff nurse grade as a diploma holder or from the nursing officer grade as a graduate. The purpose of the front-line nurse-manager's job, according to the Ghana Health Service (GHS) job description (2006), is to take a lead role in the assessment, planning, implementation and evaluation of nursing care in the unit in accordance with required standards; and to ensure management of human and material resources for nursing service delivery in the unit. The front-line nurse-managers' job, however, has become more dynamic and challenging in recent times, especially with the advent of the National Health Insurance Scheme (NHIS) that has compounded the issue of increased workload and the dwindling number of qualified nursing professionals.

Front-line nurse-managers need to actively engage in formal planning to be able to deal effectively and efficiently with their work environment for positive results. For planning to be effective, it must be formal, reflect the strategic goals of the hospital as adapted in the specific context of the unit. Planning must also be done collectively with colleagues in order to respond to individual sentiments. The planning process offers a well-structured and rational way of solving existing or future challenges within the nursing unit. Planning at the unit level is basically ad hoc and informal that normally comes up after meetings with nursing administration in most health care facilities.

It is not uncommon to observe that events often expose poor or no planning by nurse-managers in the unit, resulting in undue shortages of emergency drugs or essential materials and equipment, or a shortage of nursing staff or an unbalanced mix of skills in shifts. In some instances, the essential drugs and/or equipment may be available in the unit but are locked up in a cupboard or office and the key is with the nurse-manager who may be off duty. Operational planning at the unit level has tended at best to be informal, yet this has attracted little or no comment from nurse leaders and scholars.

The Roles of Nurse-managers

Nurse-managers can greatly influence the success of healthcare facilities because of their management role, especially at the unit level. The role of the nurse-manager is currently seen as one of the hardest, most complex roles in healthcare (Thrall, 2006). Sanders, Davidson and Price (1996) emphasize that the nurse-manager is responsible for translating strategic goals and objectives formulated at the operational level into practice; thus, the position of the nurse-manager requires an ability to interpret general concepts and integrate them into specific clinical and management performance, while simultaneously determining and monitoring outcomes.

The front line nurse-manager, formerly known as the head nurse, is a registered nurse (RN) responsible for the 24 hours business and clinical operations of a particular nursing unit. The roles of the nurse-manager according to the GHS job description (2006), are to provide leadership for the nursing team in the unit; organise and manage nursing care in the unit; ensuring that patients are treated with respect and dignity at all times; promote practice that is sensitive to the needs of patients from multi-cultural backgrounds; supervise nurses and other staff in the unit and assess their training needs to upgrade their skills.

Nurse-managers (NMs) are to investigate incident reports on patient care and safety and counsel staff accordingly; ensure maintenance of a safe and therapeutic environment for patient care within the unit; ensure maintenance of inventory of specialized items and ensure items are available at all times. Additionally, NMs are to ensure proper documentation on nursing care activities in the unit; ensure that the planning, delivery and evaluation of care programmes address the changing needs of patients in the unit; ensure the availability of the right skill mix for the delivery of nursing care during every shift; and promote the rights of both patients and nurses in the unit. NMs are to protect all confidential information concerning patients obtained in the course of professional practice and make disclosures only with the patient's consent or when disclosure can be appropriately justified. The NM carries out other assignments delegated by the Departmental manager/Head of Nursing. Above all, NMs have to balance available resources with the needs of patients and staff to ensure the best possible outcomes (GHS, 2006).

The nurse-manager's job functions falls within five areas: personnel, quality, service, business growth and financial solvency. An effective nurse-manager is flexible, consistent and approachable. She/he encourages shared decision making, ensuring that staff nurses have a voice in decisions that have an impact on their daily practice. A nurse-manager supervises direct care and clinicians, reports to a nursing director, and is a colleague to other health care managers who oversee areas such as radiology and pharmacy.

The front-line nurse-manager is seen as the chief executive officer of the clinical area; she/he works collaboratively with other managers to develop processes and procedures that ensure patient care that reflects the organization's mission and values (Schweiger, 2000). Nurse-managers coordinate patient services, conduct administrative work and handle paperwork pertaining to patients' medical records, department budgets and disciplinary actions against staff. Nurse-managers must possess strategic management skills in order to establish quality patient care as well as clinical capability across all aspects of healthcare. Nurse-managers must therefore be visionary and be able to evaluate their environment for opportunities whilst avoiding the threats in order to ensure that both staff and clients become satisfied with healthcare services.

With the advent of the title 'nurse-manager,' the role over the last decade has expanded to include financial obligations (Eiloart & Field, 1998); this however, has not been the practice of front-line nurse-managers in Ghana, especially those in the districts and regional hospitals. Ingersoll et al. (1999) concede that the responsibilities and roles of nurse-managers have not been clearly identified or described, which seem to increase the role conflict, isolation and insecurity of nurse-managers. In Ghana, however, these roles have been clearly articulated in the GHS (2006) job description, but to the authors knowledge, these roles have not been duly communicated to nurse-managers. The roles are quite numerous and affirm the statement by Hyrkas et al. (2005) that management in nursing has become increasingly demanding.

According to Cipriano (2010), nurse-managers work together to address emerging trends, adopt innovative ideas, and work toward the shared goals of quality, efficiency, and excellence in practice. The front-line NMs guide and lead nurses while contributing to the success of the healthcare facility. Furthermore, nurse-managers translate and promote organizational goals to staff and remove barriers that could hinder their performance; execution of these roles nevertheless demands effective planning.

The significance of the nurse-manager's work has never been questioned but it has been noted that the failure to actively use her/his expertise in nursing may represent a missed opportunity (Furåker & Berntsson, 2003). Many nurse-managers wish to spend more time at the bedside of the patient but understand that it is impossible to function effectively at the same time as a responsible and accountable manager. The expert nurse-manager must plan well to integrate that expertise in both management and clinical nursing.

Globally, the nurse-managers' roles have more similarities than differences. Nurse-managers in Africa, Asia and the Middle-East are balancing their nursing, educational (Bezeuidenhout et al., 1999) and managerial activities (Malan & Muller, 1997). The entire healthcare system is changing and nurse-managers play a key role in the pursuit of cost-effectiveness (Wong, 1999) and in trying to develop the model of patient-centred care and empower the nursing staff (Brandi & Naito, 2006). While the style of leadership has an effect on job satisfaction, staff retention and productiveness (Chiok Foong Loke, 2001; Dehghan Nayeri et al., 2006), nurse-managers are expected to focus more on their management roles rather than their nursing roles (Drach-Zahavy & Dagan, 2002). The nurse-manager therefore should devote more time to planning in order to anticipate the future and to contribute productively top-quality patient care.

According to Casida and Parker (2011), nurse-managers primarily comprise experienced and highly educated (80 % have baccalaureate or master's degrees) leaders who regularly attend (84 %) continuing leadership training. Ohman (2000) realized that years of experience and educational levels beyond baccalaureate degrees are antecedent variables that can positively influence nurse-managers to become transformational leaders. In Ghana, many nurses over the last few years have had at least university education and this had rather mixed outcomes which have not been measured yet.

In a descriptive study to explore nurse-managers' perception of their roles, Baxter (1993) using Mintzberg's (1973) theoretical framework, reported that nurse-managers are most familiar with roles such as monitor, disseminator, entrepreneur, disturbance handler, resource allocator, leader and liaison. Westmoreland (1993) using symbolic interactionism framework identified three role perspectives: (1) the nurse self which acknowledges patient care as self affirmation, nursing as personal development, and patient care as strategy, (2) the nurse-manager self recognises nursing management as stress and differentiation and (3) the career self, sees career as personal growth and satisfaction, and career choice as reflection of relationships, opportunity, and personal needs.

Persson and Thylefors (1999) stated that the nurse-manager role is associated with seven managerial tasks; planning, supervision, consideration, administration, organizational development, patient and research and other functions. Nurse-managers regard providing a good environment for patients as a positive aspect of their work (Gould et al., 2001) whereas the day-to-day work of caring for patients is regarded to be first priority (Skytt et al., 2008). The GHS (2006) job description of the nurse-manager clearly outlines all these roles for the nurse-manager.

Cowley (1995) acknowledged a growing tendency for learning in the workplace to be viewed as a managerial function rather than as a responsibility of educationists. The nurse-managers' key role then is to actively enhance learning by recognizing learning opportunities and helping the staff to put their learning into practice (Currie et al., 2007; Sambrook, 2007). Individual learning is a crucial element for organizational learning and nurse-managers must promote collaborative learning which requires effective knowledge-sharing practices from managers and staff members (Clarke & Wilcockson, 2001; Nutley & Davies, 2001). Effective knowledge sharing occurs through informal methods such as mentoring, team work, and informal discussions but it also needs communities of practice. For example, Dopson and Fitzgerald (2006) observed that appropriate forums for sharing knowledge locally are often lacking or are poorly integrated into the organizational and clinical routines. Most of these informal discussions can be observed in many of our facilities and students of University of Ghana have been urged to ask questions during clinical practice. This would allow nurse-managers to have an experiential learning environment for students, which would enrich their clinical experience.

Viitanen et al. (2007) studied first-line nurse-managers' work in university hospitals and found that a prominent part of the manager's job was the nurturing role (looking after staff well-being and coping), and the administrative role (human resource management, coordination and follow-up). The nurse-manager's role is without doubt very important. To be successful, therefore, the nurse-manager must engage in serious planning to become comfortable with his or her environment and not be taken by surprise in the internal and external environment.

Theoretical Basis of Planning

Existing literature on planning has four major theoretical models: comprehensive rational planning, transactive planning, incremental planning and mixed scanning (Mitchell, 2002). Comprehensive rational planning is described as instrumental rationality for analysing and making decisions (Larsen, 2003). Fainstein and Fainstein (1996) admit that the environment becomes controllable by using scientific knowledge and modern technologies, and change is engineered from the top.

The planner is considered as a 'homo economicus': he collects and analyses all necessary data with his scientific knowledge and experience to identify the common public interest; identify all possible options; evaluate them against specific criteria and thus choose the best solution (Fainstein & Fainstein, 1996; Larsen, 2003; Mitchell, 2002). The theory is centralistic, consisting of six successive steps connected by feedback loops which create the possibility of incorporating changes as a result of new information or experiences. Several modeling and analysing techniques are used, especially quantitative analyses (Larsen, 2003; Mitchell, 2002) however, the process gives no consideration to any involvement of the public (Kinyashi, 2000). This type of planning may not be appropriate for nursing units as it excludes the inputs of some stakeholders in the unit, especially the clients.

The transactive planning model is based on communicative rationality; namely communication and dialogue between planners and the people affected by planning. It is decentralised, hence, the expertise of the planner and the experimental knowledge of the population are combined and transformed into shared measures. The process is characterised by interpersonal dialogue and mutual learning, with a central focus on individual and organisational development, partnership building, and incorporation of traditional knowledge (Larsen, 2003; Mitchell, 2002). This model can be utilized by nurse-managers for the effective running of the unit.

Incremental planning is the most widely used alternative to comprehensive rational planning. Planning is considered less a scientific technique than a mixture of intuition and experience in reality (Larsen, 2003). The model describes the real everyday life in planning rather than the comprehensive rational model which perceives that there is not a right solution as resources and mental capabilities of the planners are inadequate (Kinyashi, 2006; Mitchell, 2002). The planner is therefore, considered to be a 'bounded' rational being who simplifies the complex world to an easier model rather than the best one. Planning is decentralised with both the population and more agencies involved. There is no clear determination of goals and objectives; rather, they are determined by a mixture of intuition, experience, rules of thumb and a series of consultancies (Larsen, 2003). Only a few options are considered and evaluated and a satisfying solution is selected by substantive consensus. The process becomes an ongoing chain of incremental decisions (Mitchell, 2002). This model is very typical for many nurse-managers who would normally evaluate previous work done and those outstanding in order to plan for the upcoming period.

The mixed scanning model tries to merge the strengths of the rational planning and incremental planning models and eliminate the weaknesses. The planner is considered a 'bounded' rational being, and reduces the complexity of the world to an easier model in which he or she considers few solutions in greater detail. Planning is more decentralised, with objectives and incremental decisions made in consultation with civil society (Kinyashi, 2006; Mitchell, 2002). The nurse-manager must know these theories and adapt them to resolve issues of the unit effectively.

Collective planning is more appropriate for nursing units in order to ensure commitment of nursing staff within the unit; this would bring about "we-feeling" within the unit. Thus, the mixed scanning and the incremental models can be developed as a thought-programme for nurse-managers to enable them to plan effectively. At the University of Ghana, our students are specifically given practical and theoretical knowledge in planning to enable them to plan better after graduation. Two management courses are taught in the final year of the undergraduate programme to prepare them for this task.

Planning Practices and the Nurse-Manager

The idea of planning is very relevant in any situation where there is ambiguity. Planning is that professional practice that specifically seeks to connect forms of knowledge with forms of action in the public domain. Planning is a basic function of management, and it is the principal duty of all managers. It is a systematic process and requires knowledgeable activity based on sound managerial theory (Russell, 2002). The first element of management defined by Fayol is planning, which makes a plan of action to provide for the foreseeable future. This plan of action must have unity, continuity, flexibility, and precision. Planning, according to Fayol, improves with experience, gives sequence in activity, and protects a business against undesirable changes. Fayol states that planning facilitates wise use of resources and selection of the best approaches for achieving objectives. Planning facilitates the art of handling people but planning also requires moral courage to succeed. Effective planning requires continuity of tenure and good planning is a sign of competence (Russell et al., 2002).

The GHS job description has clearly outlined planning as an essential role of the nurse-manager. It is therefore essential for the nurse-manager to be given formal training in planning in order to avoid instances where the nurse-manager and close allies meet and decide on how to manage the ward, with the other staff members excluded, as is normally seen in our wards. Rather, collective planning should be advocated for optimal outcomes that are based on the commitment and confidence of staff members. Students of UG, are encouraged to engage all staff in planning and to respect all ideas that are suggested during decision making. Each member of staff is important and should be valued; this can easily be achieved through their involvement in the formal planning process.

Formal planning calls for an explicit process for determining the running of the unit. It is a systematic process used to gain the commitment of those who are affected by the plan. Formal planning, therefore, reflects the dynamic nature of the environment (Robbins et al., 2007). The process of formal planning has identifiable guidelines, according to Cherie et al., (2005) that provide a general pattern of rational planning, namely:

1. Situation Analysis

Situational analysis helps identify the unique strengths, weaknesses, opportunities and threats of the nursing unit. Planning utilizes analysis of the past, current and future forces that affect the nursing unit. The expectations of outside interests such as government officials, health insurance companies and consumers (clients) and inside interests such as nurses, doctors, administrators and other staff are sought. The environment, demographics, available resources, legal and techno-logical factors are also considered in determining what the priorities of the nursing unit are for effective planning. Critical thinking about the past, present and future state of affairs helps in developing and implementing a well-formulated plan that is sensitive to the needs of the institution, personnel and clientele.

2. Establishment of Objectives

The specification of objectives is a major aspect of formal planning. The objectives should be written clearly, should start with the ultimate goals for the organization and be translated into specific, measurable objectives written in terms of outcome rather than action. Objectives should be challenging and able to motivate employees and improve performance.

3. Involve Management and Staff

Involving a greater number of staff results in better plans and more widespread acceptance of objectives. Cherie et al., (2007) emphasized that it is not sufficient to develop plans; plans are frequently ignored, other times they are used to rationalize a course of action previously decided. Formal planning must therefore be collective to ensure commitment to the plan.

4. Development of Alternatives

Managers usually consider many alternatives for a given situation, but a viable alternative suggests a proposed course of action that is feasible, realistic and sufficient (Cherie et al., 2005).

5. Evaluate Alternatives

Formal planning calls for an unambiguous method for evaluating the various alternatives. First, the various alternatives have to be filtered to ensure that they are within the unit's constraints. The feasible strategies should then be rated against each of the listed objectives. Various procedures can be used, such as checklists, the Delphi technique (with internal experts), or the "devil's advocate" (where one person is given the role of challenging a proposed strategy). Traditional meetings, as commonly used in informal planning, are seldom adequate (Armstrong, 2010).

6. Communication of Plans

Effective communication at all levels before performance mirrors expectations. Plans are documented to give employees direction. Managers communicate plans in two categories. First, standing plans which are used continuously to achieve consistently repeated objectives and take the form of policies, procedures and rules; secondly, plans that are used only once to achieve unique objectives such as projects, programmes, budgets, and schedule.

7. Monitoring and Evaluation of Results

Evaluation is conducted to determine whether the implemented solutions are effective in achieving the goals and also deal with evaluation of the environment for possible changes that might have rendered the solutions less effective, more effective or irrelevant (Lawrie et al., (2006). This step may begin with development of an evaluation plan well before evaluation, and development of ongoing monitoring methods to be used to continuously identify and assess the intended and unintended consequences of implementation actions.

Nurse-managers must be both visionary and operational to effectively advance nursing and to fully meet patient and facility needs. The role of front-line managers has undergone a significant development over the last few decades, moving from a traditional focus on routine supervision to that of 'mini-general manager' with responsibility for a much broader range of business management activities (Hutchinson & Purcell, 2003; Hales, 2005, 2006, 2007). This 'role evolution' of the nurse-manager is largely in response to changes in the healthcare industry and, increasingly, characteristics for success in the marketplace are based on competencies that require sophisticated business knowledge and skills (Kleinman, 2003).

To accomplish the variety of tasks required as part of the job, nurse-managers must embrace effective planning techniques. According to Diers et al. (2000) and Effken et al. (2009) frontline nurse-managers make up the largest number of operational managers in any hospital and they are the centre of action. They take on many more responsibilities to meet the numerous organizational priorities. The importance of the roles that nurse-managers collectively play in hospitals cannot be over-emphasized and cannot be compared to the role of any other single professional. Lin and Wu et al. (2007) share this view, describing the nurse-managers' role in the hospital as pivotal, influencing hospital strategy and planning activities to cope with the competitive healthcare environment. Earlier researchers such as Aroian et al. (1997) assert that nurse-managers are regarded as one of the most important assets of a hospital.

Nurse-managers use or control the use of most of the healthcare resources. The manner in which nurse-managers plan the utilization of these resources is therefore integral to ensuring efficiency in any healthcare organization. Effken et al. (2009) explain that nurse-managers are expected to identify problems or trends, design and implement innovations that will help the unit achieve targeted patient outcomes while decreasing costs to increase efficiency. Nurse-managers therefore need to understand and effectively use the planning function of managers (Marriner-Tommey, 2009).

However, the nurse-manager's knowledge and/or practice of formal planning in the unit are actually an issue of deep concern and have unfortunately not received the needed scholarly attention. In a study reported by Rakson (2010), most nurses used their time inappropriately. Effken et al. (2009) seem to agree with this assertion and acknowledge that novice nurse-managers follow a step-by-step linear process whereas expert nurse-managers take shortcuts. They claim that in expert decision making, the outcomes are not preplanned but solutions are simply pulled out of a memory bank (Effken et al., 2009). But Maison et al. (2000) disagree, saying no management action, however small, should be embarked upon without some thought and planning.

Marquis and Huston (2005) and Salehi et al. (2007) noted that nurse-managers should know the planning process and standards and use them in the working situation. Cherie et al. (2005), underscoring the need for nurses to plan, emphasize that nursing service operation in even a small agency is immensely complicated, and that careful planning, therefore, is needed to avoid waste, confusion and error. The need for effective planning in the unit cannot, therefore, be over-emphasized as this will certainly enhance efficiency, improve staff motivation and morale and also improve patient outcomes. Planning for developing quality of services and effective expenses is an important skill in nursing, (Salehi et al. 2007). Unfortunately, however, research that addresses the issue of planning in nursing management and administration is limited. The majority of the nursing literature that addresses planning relates to the clinical nursing process at the expense of the planning function of the nurse-manager.

Benefits of Planning

Hill (2004) noted that the nurse-manager clearly has enormous responsibility to sustain quality, safety, innovation, efficiency and financial performance at the unit level and to assure that staff are prepared and capable of delivering the complex patient care required. The constant demand involved in executing this broad scope of responsibility takes its toll on nurse-managers. This role consequently, must come with some fundamental planning to allow nurse-managers to be comfortable with their environment and be able to take effective charge with positive results. Nurse-managers should be empowered with planning skills to analyse environmental factors that influence the activities of the unit.

The principles of organization theory hold that planning before action improves the quality of most actions. Planning is an important precursor to action because it provides a framework within which subsequent action takes place (Ansoff, 1991), thereby facilitating the achievement of goals. Delmar and Shane (2003) asserted that planning provides three benefits: (a) it facilitates faster decision making by identifying missing information without first requiring the commitment of resources; (b) provides tools for managing the supply and demand of resources in a manner that avoids time-consuming bottlenecks; and (c) identifies action steps to achieve broader goals in a timely manner.

Abraham et al. (1999) reported that planning of specific preparatory actions may enhance the prediction of behaviour among intenders. Thus deductively, planning promotes analytical and reflective thinking culminating in predictive behaviour. Modern managers are faced with a situation in which change is the only 'constant' on which they can 'rely'. The difficulty is to decide what these changes will be, and it can be argued that it is only by planning that the nature of the changes taking place can be fully charted and understood. Managers take into account possible changes in deciding a course of action, in the form of contingency plans.

Planning is necessary in order to implement purposeful change effectively, as well as to respond to the increasing complexities and changes in the internal and external environment. In today's competitive climate, with its shrinking resources, planning has become essential for establishing a posture for the future, appropriately allocating resources, and increasing the chances of success (Jernigan, 2000). Without planning, the efforts of the unit may not be well co-ordinated. Daily routines can lead to the future being forgotten if everybody is too busy to consider medium- or long-term challenges (Hannagan, 2002). Therefore, collaborative effort and effective planning in the management of the unit is crucial.

It can be argued that planning is a rational form of management which enables organisations to acquire greater control over their future development. In the past, scientific management, by emphasizing the codification of routine tasks, encouraged the planning of operations. Jelinek (1979) argues that the equivalent of Taylor's work-study methods in terms of strategy is a system of planning and control to establish a pattern which is not overwhelmed by operational details. Marquanett (1990) acknowledged that it is the responsibility of planning to make sure that the entire organisation is fully aware of what its consumers' requirements are, the changing direction of consumer needs and consumer expectations, how technology is moving and how competitors serve their consumers. The nurse-manager therefore works in an environment of stimulus-response and should develop in his/her work a clear preference for action.

Wong (1998), in her case study of nurse-managers as a professional-managerial class, found that whereas department operation managers spend most of their time (41 %) in the areas of planning and quality improvement, ward-managers spend less time (10.0 %) performing those tasks. Planning is essential to every manager's work regardless of the level, as it provokes critical analysis of usage of resources, behaviour and performance. Having plans in the unit helps structure activities and leads to effective control of the unit. But formal plans should be flexible to avoid rigidity and encourage spontaneity and creativity.

Factors Influencing Planning

Factors within and without an organization can affect managerial planning either positively or negatively as fail-proof planning is not known to exist, but taking steps to mitigate the negative effects of these factors can ensure huge success in planning (Cliffs, 2012; Norman et al., 2008). Numerous factors have been found to affect planning.

The financial ability of the organization may negatively affect a manager's ability to plan. Norman et al. (2008) suggest that when sudden downturns occur in the organization's financial capacity, planning must be stopped, adjusted or taken in a new direction. Ghani et al. (2010) concede that training is the key to empower managers with the ability to plan. Norman et al. (2008) argue that some managers are not successful planners since they lack training and may have never been taught how to plan. When these types of managers take the time to plan, they may not know how to conduct planning as a process.

In addition, Cliffs (2012) identified commitment to the planning process as a key factor influencing the success or failure of planning. The development of a plan demands hard work and most importantly teamwork (Ghani et al., 2010). Cliffs (2012) asserted that it is much easier for a manager to claim that he/she has too much work or does not have the time to work through the required planning process than to actually devote time to developing a plan. According to Norman et al. (2008) and Cliffs (2012), another possible reason for lack of commitment towards planning is fear of failure; consequently managers sometimes tend to do little or nothing to help in the planning process.

Furthermore, the Health System Intelligence Project (2006) singled out over-reliance on overall organizational plans to the detriment of tactical and operational planning. But Cliffs (2012) counsels that the overall organizational plans (strategic plans) are aids in planning for tactical or operational managers and should be used only as such. Formulating the plan is still the manager's responsibility.

To plan successfully, managers need to use effective communication, acquire knowledge of the planning process, and solicit the involvement of others. Work environments that provide access to information, resources, support and the opportunity to learn and develop are empowering, and enhance employees' power to accomplish work through effective planning (Kanter, 1993). The health system today needs nurse-managers who are creative, able to think critically and analytically, able to resolve challenges they encounter, and who have a high mental capacity. Since the majority of the time spent at the management level is in making decisions, the ability to use the problem-solving process has a very important place in professional nursing implementation (Terzioglu, 2006).

Organizational support for nurse-managers from their supervisors is crucial to job satisfaction. Bunsey et al. (1991) highlighted the importance of supervisors' support of the manager's autonomous use of time, and suggest that support be provided for other aspects of managerial activities as well. The concept of support includes providing emotional support and allowing the front-line manager to be heard. Support was examined as a determinant in two studies and found to be positively and significantly related to nurse-managers' job satisfaction (Laschinger et al., 2006).

Having an agreed set of competencies for nurse-managers is significant. A compendium of role competencies can provide the basis for programmes of orientation focused on ensuring that nurse-managers can capably demonstrate the knowledge, skill and abilities of each competency. Skilled know-how is always situated: the nurse-manager must be able to see what is salient in a particular situation in order to draw on relevant knowledge and respond in ways that are effective (Benner et al., 2010). Since the nurse-manager works primarily through others, accurately reading a situation to grasp what is most relevant and urgent is a necessary prerequisite for determining the correct interventions. Recognizing the nature of the situation is at the heart of practical reasoning and situated cognition (Lave & Wenger, 2006).

A study by Tumulty (1992) finds that nurse-managers have too much responsibility but lack authority. Conflicts could arise if the managers have to choose between their own and others' perception of what their roles are or if they experience dissatisfaction or lack of support from staff or superiors (Skytt et al., 2008). Coulson and Cragg (1995) found that conflicts arose when nurse-managers did not get the expected support from the staff, superiors and others. Unclear expectations as well as different perceptions of the nurse-manager's roles are likely to affect the manager's performance and the staff expectations (Skytt et al., 2008).

Furthermore, the reflective and supportive characteristics of peer supervision promote the individual development and leadership of the nurse-manager. It can be concluded that peer supervision promotes quality management in nurse-managers' work (Hyrkäs et al., 2003). Poor leadership and management styles; impatience, defensive, unsupportive leadership; lack of supervision and guidance; control; and lack of recognition of contributions have been identified as major stressors (Jinks et al., 2003; Olofsson et al., 2003) to the work of the nurse-manager. On the other hand, positive workplace management initiatives such as shared organizational goals, learning opportunities, career development, reward schemes, autonomy, participation and empowerment strategies, employee health and well-being programmes, job satisfaction, and open management styles that are consistent with transformational leadership foster healthy, staff-focused workplaces (Thyer, 2003; Aust & Ducki, 2004; Joffres et al., 2004; Jooste, 2004; Park et al., 2004).

Structural empowerment indicates that a manager has the resources to meet the needs of the unit and staff, while psychological empowerment refers to congruence between the values and direction of the manager and the healthcare organization (Laschinger et al., 2004). Providing support and resources to managers can create empowerment and allow managers to use their power to positively influence unit, staff and patient outcomes. If managers are not careful, they may inadvertently leave staff feeling lost or abandoned (Vivar, 2006).

Studies of business performance suggest supervisor participation correlates with several, organizational outcomes. Maylett and Riboldi (2007) reported manager communication as significantly associated with worker engagement as well as organizational performance, including turnover, customer satisfaction, profitability and return on investment. Using a business simulation, Johnson et al. (2007) examine the influence of manager leadership on workers and acknowledge a positive relationship between leader communication, employee commitment and financial performance. Schuttler's (2008a, 2010) model of organizational performance suggests that supervisor leadership and communication directly correlate with employee performance. Sellgren et al. (2006) note that individuals perceived to be 'super' nurse-managers had more creative work climates and employees with high job satisfaction.

Challenges of the Nurse-Manager

Over the last decade management in nursing has become increasingly demanding (Hyrkas et al., 2005). Nurse-managers have taken on more administrative tasks and play a key role in achieving organizational goals of delivering high quality care to satisfy patients, creating a positive work environment that fosters staff satisfaction (McGuire & Kennerly, 2006) and, organizational resource management. When these factors are considered alongside increased patient acuity, nursing shortages and organizational pressures, questions about the scope of effective planning arise. Carney (2009, p. 413) observes that the 'different interpretations of what leadership in nursing means' raise many questions. Thus, if nurse-managers are poorly prepared for both clinical and administrative roles then the potential for planning shall increasingly be eroded.

Wilson (2005) acknowledges that formal education and support are needed for nurse-managers to effectively function in their role in the current healthcare environment. Anecdotally, many nurse-managers assume their position is based on expertise in clinical roles with little required in terms of managerial and/or leadership skills. Effective functioning in the management role, however, requires knowledge and skills related to financial management, human resource management, collective bargaining, communication and quality management. There is also additional demand for a nurse-manager to function as a transformational leader who translates vision, goals and purpose to staff at the unit level. Operating as a manager and a leader requires ongoing development of critical thinking skills and the inclination to use those skills (Zori & Morrison, 2009). Yet many nurse-managers receive little or insufficient education and support for the management role (Wilson, 2005) thus, nurse-managers are accustomed to day-to-day administration of the unit without developing plans for efficient resource management.

According to Hall et al. (2006), although the nursing community agrees on the importance of planning in nursing, there is little coordination in the application of evidence-based planning to practice. The lack of readily available evidence-based planning tools that support organizations and nurse-managers in effective planning has been a major shortcoming.

Hill (2004) noted that the nurse-manager clearly has enormous responsibility to sustain quality, safety, innovation, efficiency and financial performance at the unit level and to assure that staff are prepared and capable of delivering the complex patient care required. Additionally, the health reforms in the 1990s in Ghana dramatically changed the role of the nurse and the nurse-manager, such that the nurse-manager's responsibilities for the unit's personnel, economics of the unit and quality of patient care increased. During the last few years, many studies have explored other roles of the nurse-manager but planning of nurse-managers is conspicuously absent. Hence, the absence of evidence-based planning practices in nursing.

Planning is widely acknowledged to have numerous benefits and is so fundamental to management that it cannot be excluded from the functions of the organization. However, many healthcare managers, according to Ansah Ofei (2011), use informal plans for the management of their facilities. Duncan et al. (1996) reiterate that informal plans are equally effective and are used by a dominant leader in a stable environment. Are nurse-managers then dominant leaders or do all nurse-managers work in an uncompetitive environment? Or are nurse-managers simply interested in the day-to–day management of activities in their unit and therefore prefer informal plans?

The GHS (2006) job description has several responsibilities for the nurse-manager such as personal and people development, management, research, communication and working relationships, health safety and quality assurance apart from the main duties and responsibilities for the unit. This rather makes the roles of nurse-managers in Ghana quite challenging and stressful. Out of all the numerous responsibilities outlined, planning is essential and goes beyond the boundaries of the unit. The concept of planning has its own knowledge, skills and attitudes that have to be taught and learned but many nurse-managers are promoted to the position without any prior training in management. For someone to be comfortable with planning and lead others to plan, she or he must be knowledgeable in the principles of planning.

Planning is unarguably difficult but there is indeed so much to achieve that it is paramount that all nurse-managers come up with effective plans in line with organizational goals. These plans must be realistic, timely, measurable and relevant. Although, Koivula (2008) asserts that nurse-managers perceived lack of time for planning as a major challenge, nurse-managers must be encouraged to plan.

Conclusion

In conclusion, the roles of nurse-managers are numerous and challenging, Nurse-managers, therefore, would need all the support and effective plans to ensure organizational effectiveness and efficiency. The level of education has a direct impact on nurse-managers' knowledge and practice of planning. In-service training on planning and management with support from both management and staff are the principal necessities for effective planning at the unit level.

Planning is essential to every manager's work regardless of the level, as it provokes critical analysis of usage of resources, behaviour and performance. Having plans in the unit helps structure activities and leads to effective control of the unit but formal plans should be flexible in order to avoid rigidity and encourage spontaneity and creativity.

Reference

Ansoff, I. (1991). Critique of Henry Mintzberg's @ the Design School: Reconsidering the Basic Premises of Strategic Management. *Strategic Management Journal*, 12(6): 449-461.

Armstrong, J. (1982). The Value of Formal Planning for Strategic Decisions: Review of Empirical Research. *Strategic Management Journal*, 3(3): 197-211.

Azaare, J. . (2011). The Nature of Leadership Style in Nursing Management. *British Journal of Nursing*, 20(11): 672-80.

Beduz, M. A., Vincent, L. & Pauze, E. (2009). *Building Capacity in Nursing Human Resource Planning: A Best Practice Resource for Nursing Managers. The Nursing Human Resource Planning Best Practice Toolkit Project.* Health Force.

Bezeuidenhout, M. C., Koch, S. & Netshandama, V. O. (1999). The Role of Ward Manager in Creating a Conductive Clinical Learning Environment for Nursing Students. *Curationis*, 22(3): 46-52.

Brews, P. J. & Hunt, M. R. (1999). Learning to Plan and Planning to Learn: Resolving the Planning School/Learning School Debate. *Strategic Management Journal*, 20(10): 889-913.

Burkoski, V., & J. Tepper. (2010). Nursing Health Human Resources Demonstration Projects: Creating the Capacity for Nursing Health Human Resource Planning in Ontario's Health Care Organizations. *Canadian Journal Nursing Leadership.*, 23: 51-60.

Casida, J. & Pinto-Zipp, G. (2008). Leadership-Organizational Culture Relationship in Nursing: Units of Acute Care Hospitals. *Nursing Economics*, 26(1): 7-15.

Cherie, A. & Gebrekidan, A. B. (2005). *Nursing Leadership and Management.* Addis Ababa: Ethiopia Public Health Training Initiative, Addis Ababa University.

Cherry, B. & Jacob, S.R. (2008). *Contemporary Nursing: Issues, Trends, & Management.* 4th ed. St. Louis: Mosby Elsevier.

Clancy, C. (2003). Quality Improvement: Getting to How. *Health Services Research*, 38(2): 179-2002.

Danielson, E. & Berntsson, L. (2007). Registered nurses' perception of educational preparation for professional work and development in their profession. *Nurse Education Today*, 27, 900-908.

De Vos, A.S., Strydon, H., Fouche, C.B., & Delport C.S.L. (2005). *Research at Grassroots for Social Science and Service Professions.* 3rd ed. Pretoria: Van Schaik Publishers.

Delmar, F. & Shane, S. (2003). Does business planning facilitate the development of new venture? *Strategic Management Journal*, 24: 1165-1185.

Dougherty, D. (1992). Interpretive Barriers to Successful Product Innovation in Large Firms. *Organisation Science.*, 3(2): 179-202.

Dovlo, D. & Martineau, T. (2004). *Global Health Trust.* Available at: Global Health Trust web site: http://www.globalhealthtrust.org/doc/abstracts/WG4/DovloMartineauFINAL.pdf.

Duffield, C. (1991). First-line nurse-managers: issues in literature. *Journal of Advanced Nursing.*, 16, 1247-1253.

Executive, T. A. (2011). *AONE Nurse Executive Competencies Assessment Tool.* Retrieved from http://tigercompetencies.pbworks.com/f/Nurse_Assessment_Tool.pdf.

Ford, R. (2009). Complex leadership competency in health care: towards framing a theory. *Health service Management Research.*, 22, 101-114.

Fretwell, J. (1982). *Ward Teaching and Learning: Sister and the Learning Environment.* London: Royal College of Nursing.

Hannagan, T. (2002). *Management: Concepts and Practices.* 3rd ed. England: Pearson Education Limited.

Koivola, M. & Paunonen, M. (2001). Ward Sisters' Objectives in Developing Nursing and Problems with Development. *Journal of Nursing Management.*, 9: 287-294.

Lawrie, L., Ardal, S., Butler, J. & Edwards, R. (2006). *Health System Intelligence Project. The Health Planners Toolkit.* Ontario: Queens Printer for Ontario.

Lin, M. N., Wu, J. H., Tseng, K. H., Lavler, J. J. & Vestel, K. (2007). Management Development: A study of Nurse Managerial Activities and Skills. *Journal of Healthcare Management.*, 52(3), 156-169.

Maison, Hartle & Johnson. (2000). Planning. In: Marriner-Tomey, A. (2009). Guide to Nursing Management and Leadership. 8th ed. St. Louis: Mosby Elsevier.

Marquis, B. L. & Huston, C. J. (2006). *Leadership Roles and Management Functions in Nursing: Theory and Application.* Philadelphia: Lippincott Williams & Wilkins.

Marriner-Tomey, A. (2009). *Guide to Nursing Management and Leadership.* 8th ed. St. Louis: Mosby Elsevier.

McGuire, E., & Kennerly, S.M. (2006). Nurse-Managers as transformational and transactional leaders. *Nursing Economic$,* 24(4), 179-185.

Mintzberg, H. (1994). Fall and rise of strategic planning. . *Harvard Business Review,* , 72(1), 107-114.

Mohr, D. C., Lukas, C. V. D. & Meterko, M. (2008). Predicting healthcare employees' participation in an office redesign program: attitudes, norms and behavioural control. *Implementation Science,* 3, 47.

Noyes, B. J. (2002). Midlevel Management Education. *Journal of Nursing Administration,* 32 (1): 25-26.

Ofei, A. M. (2011). Assessment of Strategic Management Practice of Malaria Control in the Dangme West District, Ghana. *Health,* 3(6) 343-356.

Ogier, M. E. (1982). *An Ideal Sister? A Study of the Leadership Style and Verbal Interactions of Ward Sisters with Nurse Leaders in General Hospitals.* London: Royal College of Nursing.

Ogier, M. E. (1989). *Working and Learning: The Learning Environment in Clinical Nursing.* London.: Scutari.

Ohman, K. (2000). The transformational leadership of critical care nurse-managers. *Dimensions of Critical Care Nursing,* 19, 46-54.

Orton, H. D. (1981). *Ward Learning Climate.* London: Royal College of Nursing.

Pembrey, S. E. (1980). *The Ward Sister - Key to Nursing.* London.: Royal College of Nursing.

Quinn, J. B. (1980.). *Strategies for change: Logical incrementalism.* . Homewood, IL.: Irwin.

Robbins, B., & Davidhizar, R. (2007). Transformational leadership in healthcare today. *The Health Care Manager,* 26: 234-239.

Robbins, S., & Coulter, M. (2007). *Management: Pearson International edition (9th ed.).* New Jersey Prentice Hall.

Runciman, P. J. (1983). *Ward Sister at Work.* Edinburgh: Churchill Lingstone,.

Salehi, S., Bahrami, M., Hosseini, S. & Akhondzadeh, K. (2007). Critical Thinking and Clinical Decision Making in Nurse. Iranian Journal of

Nursing and Midwifery Research. Available at: http://Www.Ijnmr.Mui. Ac.Ir/Index. Php/Ijnmr/Article.

Skytt, B., Ljunggren, B., Sjoden, P. & Carlsson, M. (2007). Reasons to Leave: The Motives of First-line Nurse-Managers' for Leaving their Posts. *Journal of Nursing Management*, 15: 294-302.

Skytt, B., Ljunggren, B., Sjoden, P. & Carlsson, M. (2008). The Roles of the First-line Nurse-Manager: Perceptions from Four Perspectives. *Journal of Nursing Management*, 16: 1012-1020.

Swansburg, R. C. & Swansburg, R. J. (2002). *Introduction to Management and Leadership for Nurse-Managers*. Burlington: Jones and Bartlett Publishers.

Thrall, T. (2006). Nurturing your nurse-managers. *H&HN: Hospitals and Health Networks*, 80(4), 71-74.

Wong, F. K. (1998). The Nurse-Manager as a Professional-Managerial Class: A Case Study. *Journal of Nursing Management*, 6: 343-350.

Zori, S., Nosek, L. J. & Musil, C. M. (2010). Critical Thinking of Nurse-Managers Related to Staff RNs' Perceptions of the Practice Environment. *Journal of Nursing Scholarship*, 42:3, 305-313.

Chapter Four
The Concept of Pain and Trends in Post-operative Pain Management: Implications for Nursing Practice in Ghana

Lydia Aziato

Introduction

Pain is an unpleasant sensation that causes many individuals to seek health care. There are many types of pain including post-operative pain (POP). The repercussions of inadequately managed POP could sometimes be fatal and this calls for effective POP management. This chapter focuses on POP and the implications for nursing management. The nursing implications are geared towards recommendations for evidence-based approaches and drawing inferences for context appropriate measures in Ghana. Pain assessment is not a routine component of the Ghanaian clinical context and the need for effective pain assessment and pain management are stressed. The first section examines the concept, of pain drawing from a historical perspective, especially within the context of surgery, and describes the dimensions of pain relevant to POP management. The second section discusses POP management with a focus on contemporary evidence-based measures.

The Concept of Pain
a) Definitions of Pain

A definition for pain that refers to the personal nature of pain was given by McCaffery in (1969): "Whatever the experiencing person says it is and existing whenever the person says it does" (Lewis, Heitkemper, & Dirksen, 2004 p. 132). The subjective emphasis in this definition makes it useful in the field of pain response and management because the patient could self-report a particular feeling and obtain relief from

POP (Peters, Patijn & Lamé, 2007). However, it is not all patients who can effectively communicate their pain verbally due to speech impairment, language barrier, cognitive impairment (Mac Lellan, 2006) or altered level of consciousness characteristic of the immediate post-operative period. The definition could have been "whatever the experiencing person says or 'shows' it is and existing whenever the person says or 'shows' it does". This modification could perhaps address the verbal restriction of McCaffery's definition of pain. However, there could still be a limitation for patients who are very young and those with severe cognitive impairment. In this regard, contemporary pain studies focus on groups with special needs or deficits such as the aged (Bjoro & Herr, 2008; Chibnall & Tait, 2001; DeWaters et al., 2008). However, despite the weakness identified, McCaffery's definition gives due recognition to the personal nature of pain. In this context, studies have identified pain behaviour in many cultures (Kappesser & Williams, 2002; Stotts et al., 2007) and these responses were similar to those exhibited by Ghanaian surgical patients, such as grimacing, groaning and crying (Aziato & Adejumo, 2013).

Also, pain has been identified as an unpleasant sensation as a result of tissue damage. Thus, the International Association for the Study of Pain (IASP) (1986), defined pain as "an unpleasant sensory and emotional experience associated with actual or potential tissue damage, or described in terms of such damage" (Carter, 1998 p. 86). The use of emotional and sensory experience in this definition gives an idea of the multi-dimensionality of the pain experience. It also makes reference to the unpleasantness of pain which sets the context for the need to relieve pain. However, the definition by IASP fails to bring to the fore the largely subjective nature of pain. Also, it has been documented that pain is accompanied by nociception (sensation of pain) but it can also arise without any physiological stimuli (Macintyre & Ready, 2001), a possibility which the definition fails to address. The pain experienced by surgical patients can be related to this definition because of the 'actual tissue damage' that results from surgical incision. In a previous study, POP has been related to the trauma and inflammation associated with the surgical incision. The surgical incision initiates neural, metabolic and physiological responses which could adversely affect the patient (Brown, Christo & Wu, 2004). The study acknowledges the presence of pain associated with surgical incision and therefore includes surgical patients.

The two definitions discussed above can be linked to each other because both give an idea of the abstract concept of pain – the premise of giving an unseen phenomenon defining characteristics that has helped other researchers in their work. For example, the sensory aspect of pain has been explored to describe detailed physiological processes involved in the experience of pain.

b) Historical Perspectives

The word pain comes from the Latin word *poena* which means punishment; it also means a fine or penalty (Manimala, 2006). The history of pain can be traced as far back as the early humans. This assertion can be related to the Bible in Genesis 3:16a when God declared that a woman shall experience pain during delivery. It is documented that accounts of pain were recorded on stone tablets during the period of ancient civilization. Also, pain was associated with evil, magic and demons; and was treated with pressure, heat, water and sun. During these ancient times, pain was managed by sorcerers, shamans, priests and priestesses who employed measures such as herbs, rites and ceremonies (Witte & Stein, 2009). Perhaps this accounts for the unorthodox management of pain among some cultures in contemporary times such as the use of herbs and rituals. Later, the Greeks and the Romans postulated that the brain and the nervous system contributed to the perception of pain and this was supported in the late 1400s and 1500s where the spinal cord was recognized as a pathway for the transmission of pain (Mac Lellan, 2006). Thus, in 1664, Descartes described the pathway of pain which has been used by other researchers to develop theories of pain; for example, the gate-control theory by Melzack and Wall (1965). The knowledge derived from pain theories has helped in the management of pain and POP over the years (Macintyre & Ready, 2001; McCaffery & Beebe, 1989; Watt-Watson & Donovan, 1992).

The historical discussion of pain is linked to that of surgery as POP results from surgical incision and the inflammatory response associated with surgery. Surgery was a much feared experience for patients before the discovery of anaesthesia because of intra-operative pain, POP, sepsis and the bleeding that occurred. It is documented that measures used to reduce pain in the past included bleeding, alcohol, mandragora from the mandrake plant and opium (Badoe, 2009). Bleeding reduced blood supply to the brain and it decreased sensibility such as pain perception. Alcohol was used to stupefy the patient during surgical procedures to reduce pain. Mandragora and opium caused the patients to be lethargic during surgery; however, they experienced pain and were sometimes restrained physically. Literature regarding pain indicates that several attempts were made to control pain during surgery; for example, the use of nitrous oxide, hypnotism, and compression of nerves and arteries (Sabiston & Lyerly, 1997). A historical landmark was the discovery of diethyl ether (1846) and chloroform (1847) which were able to prevent pain during surgery. The effect caused by ether was called anaesthesia and subsequently, other forms of anaesthesia such as nerve block, spinal anaesthesia, and general anaesthesia were introduced in clinical practice (Badoe, 2009; Sabiston & Lyerly, 1997). Although anaesthesia prevents intra-operative pain, studies continue to report the persistence of POP among surgical patients over the years globally (Clegg-Lamptey & Hodasi, 2005; Dahl et al., 2003; Qu, Sherwood, McNeill & Zheng, 2008).

c) Physiology and Types of Pain

Pain perception has a strong association with the nervous system because the physiological processes involved in pain transmission hinge on the nerves (Mac Lellan, 2006). The stimulation of specialized pain nerves (nociceptors) known as transduction, transmits impulses to the central nervous system for interpretation (brain and spinal cord). The pain impulses generated in the body are inhibited by natural processes in the body, for example by the effect of neurotransmitters and this process is known as modulation. The individual becomes conscious of pain as a result of brain activity and feedback mechanism. The process involved in the individual becoming aware of a painful stimulus can also be referred to as nociperception. Previous authors have described the detailed processes involved in nociception as transduction, transmission, modulation, and perception (Hawthorn and Redmond, 1998; McCaffery and Pasero, 1999). The knowledge of the processes of pain transmission and perception helps healthcare experts to give effective care to patients suffering from pain. For example, some modalities of pain treatment such as local anaesthesia or regional nerve blocks are aimed at the nerves so that the patient will not feel the pain at the areas supplied by the nerves targeted. These may be given either pre-operatively or post-operatively (Coughlin, Karanicolas, Emmerton-Coughlin, Kanbur, Kanbur, & Colquhoun, 2010; Joshi, Rawal, Kehlet, and The PROSPECT collaboration, 2011).

Multi-dimensional phenomena of pain have been described by previous authors. For example, the sensory-discriminative dimension of pain describes the intensity of pain, the location and duration of pain as well as the quality of pain such as aching, burning and shooting. The sensory-discriminative dimension of pain enables the experiencing person to isolate pain and describe the particular sensation of pain such as the experience of POP among other sensations felt. The affective-motivational dimension of pain also describes the unpleasant nature of pain and the desire to avoid or relieve the unpleasant sensation (Coll, Ameen, & Moseley, 2004; McCaffery & Pasero, 1999).

Over the years, efforts have been made by health professionals and researchers to relieve pain due to its unpleasant nature and individuals equally make personal efforts to relieve their pain sensation. Thus, pain is recognized as the most common reason why people seek healthcare (Quinlan-Colwell, 2009; Pasero, 2009). The cognitive-evaluative dimension of pain also describes the influence of the individual's cognitive appraisal of the pain which subsequently affects the behaviour or response to the pain. The cognitive-appraisal dimension of pain is also influenced by cultural values, distractions, and hypnotic suggestion. To this end, the individuality of patients regarding their cultural background comes to bear on their responses to the use of non-pharmacologic activities in the management of pain. The influence of culture on the response to pain has been demonstrated by previous researchers in other countries (Fenwick & Stevens, 2004; Lovering, 2006).

Further, there are different types of pain described by other authors linked to the duration of pain, the source and the speed of transmission of pain nerves (Watt-Watson & Donovan, 1992). Post-operative pain is considered an acute pain and it describes a physiological response that alerts the individual of a change or malfunctioning of the body. Acute pain has a brief duration, usually less than six months; and among surgical patients, acute pain is believed to subside as healing occurs after surgery. However, the surgical patient may also experience other types of pain such as chronic pain before or after surgery due to other factors other than the surgical incision. Chronic pain is the type of pain that persists for more than six months and is prevalent among cancer patients (Macintyre & Ready, 2001; McCaffery & Pasero, 1999; Wood, 2008).

Other types of pain described according to the source of the pain include cutaneous pain (when the source of pain is the skin); somatic pain (when muscles, bones, tendons, ligaments and joints are affected); and visceral pain (when internal cavities are affected) (Macintyre & Ready, 2001). Pain can also be described according to the nature of transmission via pain nerves. Thus, there is fast pain (transmitted by A-delta fibres) and slow pain (transmitted by C fibres). Other types of pain include psychogenic pain (pain due to psychological factors), phantom pain (pain from a lost body part), and neurogenic pain (pain due to a disease of the nerve) (Hawthorn & Redmond, 1998; Mac Lellan, 2006; McCaffery & Beebe, 1994). Post-operative pain can manifest as a combination of these types of pain. For example, a patient who has had a limb amputated may experience cutaneous pain due to the surgical incision, phantom pain due to the loss of the limb, and neurogenic pain because of damage to nerves during the amputation. The specific treatment modalities for the different types of pain may differ and as a result, the patient and family need accurate and detailed information to facilitate the care provided.

POP Management and Nursing Implications
a) Pain Assessment or Evaluation

Pain assessment is an important component of pain management as it directs pain management decisions and evaluates effectiveness of pain management interventions. Over the years, POP assessment and evaluation have been researched and described and pain assessment tools have been introduced in clinical practice. The Joint Commission on Accreditation of Healthcare Organizations (JCAHO) acknowledges the right of all patients to have pain assessed and managed adequately (Collins, Gullette, & Schnepf, 2004). Thus, there are several pain assessment tools which have been used and validated in many countries and care settings for all ages by previous researchers (Abu Saad, Pool & Tulkens, 1994; Chakraborty & Mathur, 2007; Li, Herr, & Pingyan, 2009; Liu, Chung & Wong, 2003; Peters et al., 2007). Pain is assessed using both complex (multi-dimensional scales that assess more than one dimension of pain) and simple (uni-dimensional scales that assess only one dimension of pain) scales. It is argued that the use of pain assessment tools enables health professionals to apply objectivity to the subjective experience of pain. Thus, pain measurement is described as an estimation or appraisal of pain according to pre-determined objective criteria such as the use of pain scales (Bryant, 2007). Also, detailed pain assessment comprises assessment of components such as location, intensity, quality, onset, duration variations, rhythms, behavioural expressions of pain, what relieves the pain, what causes or increases the pain, and effects of pain (McCaffery & Beebe, 1989). The detailed assessment of pain is useful for chronic pain as it helps in diagnosis and evaluation of treatment outcomes. Individuals who experience chronic pain are able to give a full history of their pain as they have lived with the pain for some time. Hence, there are elaborate pain assessment scales such as the McGill Pain Questionnaire (MPQ) which is considered complex, time-consuming, and mostly appropriate for research situations rather than in clinical practice. The MPQ takes 15-30 minutes to complete; and because health care organizations do not provide adequate time for comprehensive pain assessment and documentation, it is difficult to use the MPQ in clinical practice (Gould et al., 1992).

In acute POP, the pain results from a known cause such as surgical incision and the patient might not have the energy or right level of consciousness to give a full history of the pain due to the physiological effect of surgery and anaesthesia. Subsequently, pain intensity is thought to be one of the key components of pain that affects the state of health of a person and the ability of that person to perform other functions (McCaffery & Pasero, 1999). Thus, among post-operative patients, the primary aim of pain assessment is not diagnostic; hence, a detailed pain assessment may not be necessary for all patients but rather an assessment of pain intensity with simple pain assessment scales. Such simple pain intensity scales include Visual Analog Scale (VAS), Verbal Descriptor Scale (VDS), Numeric Rating Scale (NRS), and Faces Pain Scale (FPS). Also, other pain intensity scales for acute pain assessment are the body diagrams, graphic rating scales, computer graphic scales, picture scales and coin scales (Hall-Lord & Larsson, 2006). Post-operative pain assessment most commonly involves the assessment of pain intensity by the use of simple scales such as the NRS, the VAS and the VRS (Coll, Ameen & Mead, 2004). Pain assessment tools are not routinely employed in clinical practice in Ghana and it is anticipated that appropriate pain assessment tools will be developed or existing tools validated for POP assessment in Ghana.

b) Conventional POP Management

Globally, POP management has gone through myriad changes as a result of research activities in this area. In the past, post-operative pain was primarily managed with analgesics such as parenteral opioids – morphine injection (pethidine - meperidine), suppository (diclofenac – volteran or paracetamol - acetaminophen), and tablet (tramadol -ultram, paracetamol, and toradol – ketorolac tromethamine) as is current in the Ghanaian surgical context (Aziato, 2012). Post-operative analgesics such as diclofenac and paracetamol are also given in the form of suppositories. Analgesics were prescribed to be administered intramuscularly on 'as needed' (PRN - *pro re nata*) basis. However, patients continued to experience moderate to severe POP and this led to clinical studies that informed changes in the management of pain. The administration of analgesics through the intramuscular route prescribed on PRN basis are considered obsolete with the introduction of new techniques of POP management (Hofer & Högström, 1995).

Research identified the barriers to POP management that span health professionals, patients and their relations, and organizational and institutional factors. For example, health professionals give inadequate opioid analgesics post-operatively because they fear potential side effects such as addiction or respiratory depression (McCaffery & Pasero, 1999). Attempts have been made to surmount these barriers and this has led to changes in the administration of analgesics such as the use of multi-modal analgesia (Jirarattanaphochai & Jung, 2008), pre-emptive analgesia (Joshi et al., 2011), and regular around-the-clock analgesia (Paice, Noskin, Vanagunas & Shott, 2005). Attempts have been made for training and education of health professionals to enhance POP management over the years with some level of impact (MacLellan, 2004). It is also acknowledged that patient and family education is necessary to improve POP management and studies have reported the positive impact of such educational programmes (Fredericks, Guruge, Sidani & Wan, 2010).

Within the Ghanaian context, POP management with injection of pentazocine (sosegon), morphine or pethidine prescribed eight-hourly or PRN was reported. However, the sosegon injection phased out after a while and morphine use among post-operative patients was not common. Pethidine injection had remained the most common opioid analgesic among post-operative patients. The prescription of analgesics ranged from 12-hourly to 6-hourly and was ordered PRN for 24 to 48 hours (Aziato & Adejumo, 2013). Studies conducted among Ghanaian post-operative patients indicated that POP is inadequately managed (Clegg-Lamptey & Hodasi, 2005). A study of post-operative patients and surgical health professionals revealed that nurses did not administer post-operative analgesics as prescribed due to unavailability of the analgesic such as opioids, fear of addiction, and organizational laxity where health professionals were not held accountable for lapses in analgesic administration (Aziato & Adejumo, 2013).

Thus, a recent effort to improve POP management is the development of culturally appropriate clinical guidelines adopted by the Ghana Health Service. The author's PhD study adopted an innovative, rigorous, multi-step, ethnographic approach to achieve this goal. The innovative approach triangulated multiple methods of data collection such as individual interviews, clinical observation, and review of clinical documents. Multiple sources of data such as patients, health professionals, patients' family and key informants were used. The study also involved a systematic review of the current evidence of post-operative pain management. Thus, an in-depth comprehensive understanding of the context factors and the scientific evidence formed the basis of a draft clinical guideline. The draft guideline was subjected to an innovative process involving expert review, participants' review, and a consensus forum involving all relevant stakeholders for pain management such as the Ghana Health Service, WHO, health professionals, patient and family representatives, etc. The new guideline emphasizes appropriate patient and family education, effective team work among the multidisciplinary health team, input and monitoring from hospital/unit leadership, and use of contemporary, evidence-based, POP management recommendations (Aziato, 2012). Clinical guidelines have been noted to guide clinicians in their patient management decisions (Hewitt-Taylor, 2004). It is hoped that the implementation of the clinical guideline in clinical practice will enhance POP management in the near future.

c) Advanced POP Management Techniques

The persistence of ineffective POP management has resulted in the development of advanced techniques that have contributed to improvements in POP management. The contemporary advanced techniques for POP management routinely used in clinical practice in developed countries include intravenous patient-controlled analgesia (PCA) and epidural analgesia (Pasero & McCaffery, 2011). The epidural analgesia is available in two forms – continuous and patient-controlled. The PCA devices for management of POP are programmed to administer a specific amount of analgesia at a time (Pasero & McCaffery, 2007). Thus, health professionals are required to undergo specialized training to use the device properly. Patient education improves the use of PCA devices. The use of the PCA does not guarantee a pain score of zero; however, it gives the patient the needed comfort post-operatively. A patient on PCA may be given other forms of analgesics as the condition demands. Research indicates that epidural analgesia leads to better pain control than PCA although epidural analgesia is associated with a greater incidence of pruritus (Huang, Cunningham, Laurito & Chen 2001). Oral PCA is less invasive but its usage is restricted within the post-operative environment because of post-operative *nil per os* (nothing by mouth). Also, PCA can be administered through the subcutaneous, epidural and intrathecal routes. Another type of patient-controlled regional analgesia recommended for patients who undergo day-surgery involves an elastrometric balloon pump with an epidural catheter and a clamp that a patient can open and close to receive a dose of analgesic (Azad et al., 2000; Huang et al., 2001).

In addition, non-pharmacologic adjuvant measures for POP management such as transcutaneous electrical nerve stimulation (TENS), electro acupuncture, and psychological supportive therapeutic modalities such as the use of systematic relaxation have been introduced (Huang et al., 2001). It is stressed that non-pharmacologic measures of POP management should be employed in addition to analgesics since the use of non-pharmacologic measures alone are not effective in the management of POP.

In the Ghanaian clinical context, advanced techniques for post-operative pain management are not routinely employed. However, epidural analgesia is used post-operatively for patients who can afford but it is not covered by the National Health Insurance Scheme (NHIS). The average Ghanaian patient is unable to afford the cost of the epidural catheter. Also, a few private hospitals and specialized units of tertiary health facilities use advanced pain management techniques for POP management. The advanced pain management techniques are employed by anaesthetists and nurses with special training. There are inadequate numbers of anaesthetists and no specialist pain nurses in Ghana, which further hinders the use of advanced pain management techniques (Aziato, 2012). The development of patient-controlled analgesia techniques addresses the subjectivity and individuality of pain such that an individual controls his/her pain management. The PCA allows variations in analgesic requirements for post-operative patients and perhaps it is a technique that curbs the fear of health professionals about the administration of opioid analgesics. The effective application of the advanced techniques involves regular training of health professionals and effective patient education to ensure that maximum benefit is derived from the techniques (McCaffery & Pasero, 1999).

d) **Effects of Pain**

Inadequately treated acute pain has been found to affect most systems of the body -- including the cardiovascular, respiratory, gastrointestinal, neuroendocrine or metabolic and musculoskeletal systems -- as well as the psychological state of the patient. Some specific problems post-operative patients may develop include hypertension, deep vein thrombosis (DVT), infection, chronic pain, decreased gastric and bowel motility, and increased catabolic hormones such as cortisol, glucagon, rennin, and angiotensin (Hawthorn & Redmond, 1998; MacLellan, 2006; Macintyre & Ready, 2001). Some of the effects of inadequate pain management, for example DVT, can have fatal consequences. Also, inadequately managed pain can result in other problems, for example, the release of angiotensin may cause the blood pressure to rise resulting in hypertension. Nurses and other multidisciplinary team members should explain the effects of inadequate pain management to the patient to enhance early ambulation (walk or move around), rehabilitation, comfort and satisfaction. Effective pain management prevents complications and shortens hospital stay (Macintyre & Ready, 2001). When the patient understands these benefits and effects, he/she, to a large extent, will cooperate with the multidisciplinary team to achieve effective pain management.

The economic burden of pain when it is inadequately managed makes it a worldwide public health issue and it is recognized that the untoward effects of pain have economic consequences (McCaffery & Pasero, 1999). These consequences have been identified as direct cost from medical care expenditure and indirect costs from lost or reduced work output of patients and families, insurance cost, cost of retraining, and lost tax revenue. There are also intangible costs from psychological and social stress (MacLellan, 2006; Turk & Melzack, 2001). Studies have also reported the large amount of money spent on pain treatment in the USA (Turk & Melzack, 2001). Hence, the WHO and the IASP pioneered a global initiative to draw awareness to inadequately treated acute pain which contributes to delay in healing in post-operative and injured patients (Berry & Dahl, 2000).

Nursing Implications

Nurses spend more hours with the patient than other health profes-sionals and they have key roles to play in POP management. Advances in POP management techniques demand that nurses obtain further specialized training to effectively employ such techniques. Effective POP management requires effective multidisciplinary team work and this recognition has led to the establishment of acute pain teams in some developed countries that are mostly led by the anaesthesiolo-gists. When skilled nurses lead the acute pain team, it is less expensive and also leads to effective pain management outcomes (McDonnell, Nicholl & Read, 2003). This presupposes that nurses develop skills for team work and leadership to enhance their changing roles in contem-porary POP management. Research continues to report inadequate administration of opioid analgesics by nurses and it is important that nurses make a conscious effort to change their attitude towards administration of post-operative analgesics. The need for nurses to administer analgesics regularly and not wait for patients to report pain before administering the analgesic is clear. Also, nurses should make an effort to understand the concept of multimodal analgesia so that they will not administer an incomplete prescription. Nurses are required to assess pain regularly because the assessment findings guide POP management. Thus, nurses should believe the patient's self-report of pain and ensure that assessment findings are accurately documented and appropriate interventions are instituted as necessary.

Nurses are required to give adequate education to their patients. The subjective nature of pain requires the need for active involvement of patients and their relatives in pain management. Patients may harbour misconceptions about POP. For example, within the Ghanaian context, post-operative patients expect to experience pain after surgery and they do not consider that the ill-effects of POP can be detrimental to their health. Some patients also do not ask about the medications they are given because they feel that health professionals should know better what medication is best for them (Aziato, 2012). Thus, patients and their relatives should be educated to participate actively in pain management decisions and nurses should take a lead role in patient education. Without patient and family education, the introduction of advanced POP management techniques such as PCA within the Ghanaian clinical context could be a challenge. Inadequate pain control within the Ghanaian context may result from patients' expectations of pain and their fears of side effects of the drugs. The subjective nature of pain requires that when pain assessment tools are introduced for POP assessment, nurses should ensure that patients are allowed to self-report their pain.

Conclusions and Recommendations

This chapter has highlighted significant issues regarding the concept of pain and POP management. It has emphasized that the subjective nature of pain mandates active involvement of patients in pain assessment and management. Post-operative pain management involves the use of analgesics and non-pharmacologic measures which serve as adjuvants or supplements to analgesic therapy. It is essential that health professionals prescribe and administer analgesics on regular a basis rather than on a PRN basis unless the patient's condition warrants judicious assessment of other clinical factors that could indicate increased risk related to regular pain medication administration such as respiratory depression and low blood pressure. It has been established that the use of two or more different analgesics post-operatively and administering analgesics before pain occurs helps to effectively manage POP. Some advanced techniques for POP management such as PCA allow patients to be actively involved in their analgesic requirements. However, it is paramount to effectively educate patients and their relatives on POP management so that they can help achieve POP management targets. The curriculum for training nurses, for example at the undergraduate level, should be reviewed to include current recommendations on POP and emphasize core components of the new clinical guidelines.

It is recommended that health professionals acquire the requisite training in POP management including specialized training in the advanced techniques to promote better POP management outcomes. In resource-limited clinical environments such as those found in Ghana, it is recommended that effective patient education, effective team work among the multidisciplinary team, effective leadership, and incorporation of evidenced-based POP management measures such as the use of multimodal and preemptive analgesia could help to effectively manage POP. The need to develop or adapt an existing pain assessment tool and validate such tools in Ghana to assist future pain management and research is evident.

References

Abu-Saad, H. H., Pool, H. & Tulkens, B. (1994). Further Validity Testing of the Abu-Saad Paediatric Pain Assessment Tool. *Journal of Advanced Nursing,* 19, 1063-1071.

Azad, S. C., Groh, J., Beyer, A., Schneck, D., Dreher, E., & Peter, K. (2000). Continuous Peridural Analgesia vs Patient-Controlled Intravenous Analgesia for Pain Therapy after Thoracotomy. *Anaesthesist,* 49(1).

Aziato, L. & Adejumo, O. (in press). The Ghanaian Surgical Nurse and Post-Operative Pain Management: A Clinical Ethnographic Insight. *Pain Management Nursing.*

Aziato, L. (2012). *Development of Clinical Guidelines for the Management of Post-Operative Pain within the Medico-Socio-Cultural Context of Ghana.* Bellville: University of the Western Cape.

Badoe, E. A. (2009). A Brief History of Surgery. In: Badoe, E. A., Archampong, E. Q. and da Rocha-Afodu, J. T. eds. *Principles and Practice of Surgery including Pathology in the Tropics* (pp. 1-11). Tema: Ghana Publishing Corp.

Berry, P. H. & Dahl, J. L. (2000). The New JCAHO Pain Standards: Implications for Pain Management Nurses. *Pain Management Nursing,* 1(1), 3-12.

Bjoro, K. & Herr, K. (2008). Assessment of Pain in the Nonverbal or Cognitively Impaired Older Adult. *Clinics in Geriatric Medicine,* 24(2), 237-262.

Brown, A. K., Christo, P. J. & Wu, C. L. (2004). Strategies for Postoperative Pain Management. *Best Practice & Research Clinical Anaesthesiology,* 18(4), 703-717.

Bryant, H. (2007). Pain: A Multifaceted Phenomenon. *Emergency Nurse,* 14(10), 6-10.

Carter, B. (ed.). (1998). *Perspectives on Pain: Mapping the Territory.* New York: Clare Parker.

Chakraborty, A. & Mathur, S. (2007). Rupee Scale: for measurement of pain in India. 12(2), 3p.

Chibnall, J. T. & Tait, R. C. (2001). Pain Assessment in Cognitively Impaired and Unimpaired Older Adults: A Comparison of Four Scales. *Pain,* 92(1-2), 173-186.

Clegg-Lamptey, J. N. A. & Hodasi, W. M. (2005). An Audit of Aspects of Informed Consent and Pain Relief in General Surgical Units of Korle Bu Teaching Hospital. *Ghana Medical Journal,* 39(2), 63-67.

Coll, A. M., Ameen, J. R. M., & Mead, D. (2004). Postoperative Pain Assessment Tools in Day Surgery: Literature Review. *Journal of Advanced Nursing,* 46(2), 124 - 133.

Coll, A. M., Ameen, J. R. M., & Moseley, L. G. (2004). Reported Pain after Day Surgery: A Critical Literature Review. *Journal of Advanced Nursing,* 46(1), 53 - 65.

Collins, A. S., Gullette, D., & Schnepf, M. (2004). Break through Language Barriers: Is Your Pain Assessment Lost in Translation? *Nursing Management,* 35(8), 34.

Coughlin, S. M., Karanicolas, P. J., Emmerton-Coughlin, H. M. A., Kanbur, B., Kanbur, S., & Colquhoun, P. H. D. (2010). Better Late than Never? Impact of Local Analgesia Timing on Postoperative Pain in Laparoscopic Surgery: A Systematic Review and Meta-Analysis. *Surgical Endoscopy and Other Interventional Techniques,* 24(12).

Dahl, J. L., Gordon, D., Ward, S., Skemp, M., Wochos, S., & Schurr, M. (2003). Institutionalizing Pain Management: The Post-operative Pain Management Quality Improvement Project. *The Journal of Pain,* 4(7), 361-371.

DeWaters, T., Faut-Callahan, M., McCann, J. J., Paice, J. A., Fogg, L., Hollinger-Smith, L., et al. (2008). Comparison of Self-reported Pain and the PAINAD Scale in Hospitalized Cognitively Impaired and Intact Older Adults after Hip Fracture Surgery. *Orthopaedic Nursing,* 27(1), 21-28.

Fenwick, C., & Stevens, J. (2004). Postoperative Pain Experiences of Central Australian Aboriginal Women. What Do We Understand? *Aust. J. Rural Health, 12,* 22 - 27.

Fredericks, S., Guruge, S., Sidani, S., & Wan, T. (2010). Postoperative Patient Education: A Systematic Review. *Clinical Nursing Research, 19*(2), 144-164.

Gould, T. H., Crosby, D. L., Harmer, M., Lloyd, S. M., Lunn, J. N., Rees, G. A. D., et al. (1992). Policy for Controlling Pain after Surgery: Effect of Sequential Changes in Management. British Medical Journal *305,* 1187-1193.

Hall-Lord, M. L., & Larsson, B. W. (2006). Registered Nurses' and Student Nurses' Assessment of Pain and Distress Related to Specific Patient and Nurse Characteristics. *Nurse Education Today, 26*(5), 377-387.

Hawthorn, J., & Redmond, K. (1998). *Pain: Causes and Management.* UK: Biddles Ltd.

Hewitt-Taylor, J. (2004). Clinical Guidelines and Care Protocols. *Intensive and Critical Care Nursing, 20*(1), 45-52.

Hofer, S., and Högström, H. (1995). The Role of the Nurse in Post-operative Pain Therapy. *Baillière's Clinical Anaesthesiology, 9*(3), 461-467.

Huang, N., Cunningham, F., Laurito, C. E., & Chen, C. (2001). Can We Do Better With Postoperative Pain Management? *The American Journal of Surgery, 182*(5), 440-448.

Jirarattanaphochai, K., & Jung, S. (2008). Nonsteroidal Anti-inflammatory Drugs for Postoperative Pain Management after Lumbar Spine Surgery: A Meta-analysis of Randomized Controlled Trials. *Journal of Neurosurgery: Spine, 9,* 22-31.

Joshi, G. P., Rawal, N., Kehlet, H., & The PROSPECT Collaboration. (2011). Evidence-based Management of Postoperative Pain in Adults Undergoing Open Inguinal Hernia Surgery. *British Journal of Surgery, 99*(2), 168-185.

Kappesser, J., & Williams, A. C. d. C. (2002). Pain and Negative Emotions in the Face: Judgements by Health Care Professionals. *Pain, 99*(1-2), 197-206.

Lewis, S. M., Heitkemper, M. M., and Dirksen, S. R. (2004). *Medical-Surgical Nursing: Assessment and Management of Clinical Problems* 6th ed. St. Louis: Mosby.

Li, L., Herr, K., & Pingyan, C. (2009). Postoperative Pain Assessment With Three Intensity Scales in Chinese Elders. *Journal of Nursing Scholarship, 41*(3), 241-249.

Liu, J. Y. W., Chung, J. W. Y., & Wong, T. K. S. (2003). The Psychometric Properties of Chinese Pain Intensity Verbal Rating Scale. *Acta Anaesthesiol Scand 47*, 1013 - 1019.

Lovering, S. (2006). Cultural Attitudes and Beliefs About Pain. *Journal of Transcultural Nursing, 17*(4), 389- 395.

Mac Lellan, K. (2004). Postoperative Pain: Strategy for Improving Patient Experiences. *Journal of Advanced Nursing, 46*(2), 179 - 185.

Mac Lellan, K. (2006). *Management of pain.* UK: Nelson Thornes Ltd.

Macintyre, P. E., & Ready, L. B. (2001). *Acute Pain Management: A Practical Guide.* London: W.B. Saunders.

Manimala, R. (2006). Acute Post Operative Pain. *Indian Journal of Anaesthesia, 50*(5), 340-344.

McCaffery, M., & Beebe, A. (1989). *Pain: Clinical Manual for Nursing Practice.* St. Louis: Mosby.

McCaffery, M., & Beebe, A. (1994). *Pain: Clinical manual for nursing practice.* UK ed. London: Mosby.

McCaffery, M., & Pasero, C. (1999). *Pain: Clinical Manual.* London: Mosby Inc.

McDonnell, A., Nicholl, J., & Read, S. (2003). Acute pain teams in England: Current provision and their role in post-operative pain management. *Journal of Clinical Nursing, 12*, 387-393.

Paice, J. A., Noskin, G. A., Vanagunas, A., & Shott, S. (2005). Efficacy and Safety of Scheduled Dosing of Opioid Analgesics: A Quality Improvement Study. *The Journal of Pain, 6*(10), 639-643.

Pasero, C. (2009). Challenges in Pain Assessment. *Journal of PeriAnesthesia Nursing, 24*(1), 50-54.

Pasero, C., & McCaffery, M. (2007). Orthopaedic Postoperative Pain Management. *Journal of PeriAnesthesia Nursing, 22*(3), 160-174.

Pasero, C., and McCaffery, M. (2011). *Pain Assessment and Pharmacologic Management.* St. Louis: Mosby/Elsevier.

Peters, M. L., Patijn, J., & Lamé, I. (2007). Pain Assessment in Younger and Older Pain Patients: Psychometric Properties and Patient Preference of Five Commonly Used Measures of Pain Intensity. *Pain Medicine, 8*(7), 601 - 610.

Qu, S., Sherwood, G. D., McNeill, J. A., & Zheng, L. (2008). Postoperative Pain Management Outcome in Chinese Inpatients. *Western Journal of Nursing Research, 30*(8), 975-990.

Quinlan-Colwell, A. D. (2009). Understanding the Paradox of Patient Pain and Patient Satisfaction. Journal of Holistic Nursing, 27(3), 177-182.

Sabiston, D. C., & Lyerly, K. H. (1997). *Textbook of Surgery: Pocket Companion.* Philadelphia: W.B. Saunders Company.

Stotts, N. A., Puntillo, K., Stanik-Hutt, J., Thompson, C. L., White, C., & Rietman Wild, L. (2007). Does Age Make a Difference in Procedural Pain Perceptions and Responses in Hospitalized Adults? *Acute Pain, 9*(3), 125-134.

Turk, D., & Melzack, R. (2001). The Measurement of Pain and the Assessment of People Experiencing Pain. In: Turk, D. C. and Melzack, R. eds. *Handbook of Pain Assessment* (2nd ed., pp. 3-11). London: The Guildford Press.

Watt-Watson, J. H., & Donovan, M. I. (1992). *Pain Management: Nursing Perspective.* St. Louis: Mosby-Year Book, Inc.

Witte, W., & Stein, C. (2009). History, Definitions and Contemporary Viewpoints. In: Kopf, A. and Patel, N. B. eds. *Guide to Pain Management in Low Resource Settings* (pp. 7-11). Seattle: International Association for the Study of Pain (IASP).

Wood, S. (2008). Anatomy and physiology of pain. *Nursing times.net.* . Available at: http://www.nursingtimes.net/nursingpractice/clinical-zones/pain-management/anatomy-and-physiologyof-pain/1860931. article. [Accessed 12 July 2010].

Chapter Five
Road Traffic Injuries (RTIs) in Ghana: Challenges to Nursing Care
Lillian Akorfa Ohene

Introduction

In recent times, injuries are increasingly being recognized as a major public health problem. Among the leading causes of injuries is road traffic accidents (RTAs). Globally, there are an estimated 10 million motor vehicle crashes annually (Nantulya & Reich, 2002a) and nearly three-quarters of the deaths resulting from these crashes occur in low- and middle-income countries (of which Ghana is one) (Afukaar, Antwi & Ofosu-Amaah, 2003). These high rates of RTAs present one of the most daunting challenges to low-income nations, as their health systems in general are least prepared to respond (Ozgediz et al., 2009a). Noting that RTAs kill and maim people, destroy families and devastate communities in the process, this chapter discusses the events and processes that occur after a motor accident in Ghana, with particular emphasis on the nursing management of accident victims. The chapter will also compare how an accident victim is managed in Ghana with global standards, and also take a closer look at best practices in high-income countries. Our overall aim is to educate readers on the effort nurses put into managing accident victims after they arrive at a hospital, and on some challenges in managing and rehabilitating them.

It is important to note that there are various theoretical frameworks for managing accident victims at the emergency unit. Among such frameworks are; emergency nursing assessment framework (Curtis, Murphy, Hoy & Lewis, 2009).

This paper discusses the uniqueness of the emergency nursing process and practice environment in relation to other nursing and caring situations. The complexity and uncertainty surrounding emergency nursing practice requires a structured approach based on initial assessment and decision making. Such approaches include the five-step emergency nursing assessment framework (ENAF) for holistic nursing care (Olive, 2003) and Roy's adaptation model (Ingram, 1995).

The paper discusses types of road accident injuries, the realities of RTAs, responding to accident scenes, and the reception and immediate care of RTA patients at the hospital with an emphasis on nursing care. The subsequent routine care of RTA patients in hospital settings and the complications and challenges of nursing them is also presented. The paper concludes with recommendations for reducing RTAs and improving care for victims in Ghana.

Types of Road Accident Injuries

Road traffic accidents (RTAs), or simply motor accidents, are unexpected events producing unintended injuries, deaths or damage to property involving one or more vehicles on a road. RTAs may take any of the following three forms singly or in combination:

1. Fatal: where death occurs;
2. Serious: where persons sustain serious injuries and may be maimed/deformed and damage to property sometimes beyond economic repairs.
3. Minor: where persons sustain minor injuries and normally treated and discharged, with slight damage to properties.

Looking closely at the type of injuries that result from RTAs, Parry and Girotti, (2008) described the nature of vehicle collision, the location of occupants in the vehicle, and the pattern of injuries likely to be sustained. According to these authors, the collision types commonly reported are frontal impact or head-on collisions which often result in fractures and/or dislocations, particularly to the thorax. This may lead to haemothorax, pneumothorax, flail chest and blunt cardiac injury. They are also the leading causes of brain injuries and internal bleeding in most accident cases (Liberman et al. 2004).

Parry and Girotti (2008) describe lateral impact or 'T-bone' collisions as another form of traffic accident which often takes place at road intersections. It often results in cervical fractures, dislocation and or ligamentous injuries to the neck. Fractures of the clavicle (shoulder) are also common. The direct compression of the lateral rib cage may also lead to rib fractures and damage to the surrounding internal organs, (i.e. the spleen, liver and kidneys). Lateral impact often does not spare the pelvic cage, with complex fractures also occurring in the pelvic ring (Daniels & Fulcher, 1997).

There are also rear-impact collisions where the vehicle is hit from behind, causing injuries to the head and neck and commonly the cervical spine. It is argued that since the occupant is in contact with the seat of the vehicle, he or she will move forward at impact. However, the sudden extension-flexion-extension motion of the cervical spine often predisposes the victim to ligamentous damage injuries. Finally, rotational and rollover impact due to a combination of forces results in multiple injuries. Currently, there is evidence that vehicle occupants wearing seatbelts fare much better in the unfortunate event of an accident. (Nirula, Talmor, & Brasel, 2005). Effective management and control of these road traffic injuries involves multidisciplinary approach. Timely interventions and cost-effective health care management will go a long way to reduce the burden of RTAs in low- and middle-income countries since it is often the poor in society who bears the burden of RTA complications (Mock et al., 2005).

The Realities of Road Traffic Accidents

It is estimated that over 1.2 million people die each year on the world's roads and between 20 and 50 million suffer non-fatal injuries (Sauaia et al., 1995; Mayou & Bryant, 2003; Johnell & Kanis, 2004). RTAs have been recorded as the tenth leading cause of death worldwide, and the many road traffic injuries (RTIs) affect all populations, regardless of age, sex, income, or geographic region (Naci, Chisholm & Baker, 2009). Road traffic injuries are among the top three causes of death among the 5 to 44 years age group (Nantulya & Reich, 2002b; Kopits & Cropper, 2005). It is also alarming that over 90 percent of the world's road fatalities occur in low- and middle-income countries, which are estimated to have only 48 percent of the world's vehicles (Jacobs et al., 2000). It is predicted that the situation will worsen if nothing is done. For example, road accidents could become the third leading cause of death and disability worldwide by 2020 (Murray et al., 1997). The World Health Organization (WHO), also studying the trends, believes that RTIs will rise to become the fifth leading cause of death worldwide by 2030.

Road traffic injuries remain a major health issue in Ghana (Aidoo, Amoh-Gyimah & Ackaah, 2013). The national average fatality index is rated 8.5 / 100,000 population per year; with some specific figures of 21,709 injuries and 48, 605 casualties between 2005 to 2007 (Damsere-Derry, Ebel, Mock Afukaar & Donkor, 2010).

Road injuries are on the ascendency with daily media reports in Ghana.

Responding to Accident Scenes

The majority of studies of trauma and trauma management systems have been conducted in the United States followed by the European countries (Mock, Arreola-Risa & Quansah, 2003; Dolan & Holt, 2007; Dunn, Gwinnutt & Gray, 2007; MacFarlane & Benn, 2003). Some of these studies have critically examined pre-hospital care and its resultant effects on accident victims as well as the nation's medical system in general. Frequently reported from these high-income countries is the alarming death toll that occurs during transportation of accident victims to hospitals. It is documented that approximately half of all trauma deaths occurs in the pre-hospital settings (Murray et al., 1997b). This supports the assertion that increased survival of severely injured patients may be obtained by early transfer to a highly specialized care unit within a hospital (Sampalis et al., 1997). Following the increased number of studies in the area of trauma and the application of evidence-based interventions, it is not surprising to read reports that in middle- and high-income countries, integration of pre-hospital trauma life support and integrated emergency medicine and trauma care systems are responsible for a marked reduction of morbidity and mortality following trauma (Ozgediz et al., 2009b). Thus, in areas where there is an effective ambulance system that responds to emergency calls, and assists victims on their way to hospitals, decreased rates of mortality are recorded among accident cases (Cornwell III et al., 2000).

A look at trauma issues in low-income countries shows that the story is different when one considers the initial response to accident scenes and pre-hospital management. The lessons from higher income countries are that the first few minutes after an accident and the nature of medical care received are very crucial in determining the outcome of injuries. The literature shows that initial stages of care given to accident victims — which includes movement — must be conducted with conscious effort to reduce pain and prevent risk of further injury or complications (Mock, Jurkovich, Arreola-Risa, Maier, et al., 1998; Ohene, 2008). Meanwhile, a number of publications have also advocated lay person assistance at accident scenes (Razzak & Kellermann, 2002). It has been observed that in Ghana and Nigeria (and probably in other low-income countries), most accident victims are brought to hospital either by good samaritans or drivers and passengers who may have been involved in the same accident or happened to have arrived at the scene in time (Lagarde, 2007; Ohene, 2008). This implies that in most low-income countries), the first people to arrive at accident scenes are people who may lack the knowledge in first aid techniques (Mock et al., 2003). A study conducted by Ohene (2008) finds that nurses working at the accident and emergency unit of a tertiary hospital welcomed the introduction of the ambulance system in Ghana. However, participants in the study also stated that in the few instances they received emergency trauma patients from the ambulance crew, the majority of patients who came through the ambulance system were referrals from other health facilities and not directly from accident scenes. Ghana National Ambulance Service was established by the Ministry of Health in 2004 to provide first aid services en route to hospital facilities. The ambulance services, mainly operated by emergency medical technicians are believed to be functional in all the 10 regions of Ghana (Osei-Ampofo et al., 2013). The literature from Ghana and Nigeria indicate that pre-hospital trauma systems need serious attention and further expansion in order to achieve national coverage.

Reception and Immediate Care of RTI Patients at the Hospital

It is known that upon arrival at the hospital, patients believe that they are cared for by competent professionals who are experts in their field (Jacoby, Ackerson & Richmond, 2006). In most emergency units globally, nurses are the front-line caregivers at the accident trauma departments of hospitals. Throughout the 24-hour work schedule of hospitals, the nurse is always at post, ready to receive patients involved in RTA or trauma of any kind (Mckay, 2006; Ohene, 2008). The nurse, being the first member of the health team to receive accident victims, must have the requisite skills to handle RTA victims with care. Other emergency team members who come in to care for accident victims are the surgeon, orthopaedic specialist, neurologist, anesthetics, pharmacist, critical care nurse and other relevant staff such as the radiologist, laboratory personnel and physiotherapist.

After receiving the accident patient, a quick assessment is carried out by the nurse. Early stage assessment begins with assessment of the airway, breathing, circulation and pulse (ABC). According to recent studies (Mayou & Bryant 2001, Nyström 2002; McConnell, Eyres & Nightingale, 2008), rapid survey and its focus on life-saving interventions supersedes all other priorities, including the psychological and social support needs of a patient in crisis. Standards and evidence-based practices have also shown that following motor accidents, patients may be predisposed to airway obstruction commonly due to displacement of the tongue, loose teeth, impacted dentures, foreign bodies and multiple facial fractures (Brennan, 2002). The airway assessment focuses on identifying obvious causes of obstructions, the effect on mental status, abnormal inspiratory effort and altered airflow. After establishing a clear airway and breathing pattern, circulatory assessment, which aims at identifying signs of shock, follows immediately. Shock is a disease state in which oxygenation is inadequate to meet tissue metabolic requirements. The primary survey requires concurrent treatment of all three areas of priority mentioned above, hence, the nurse may often be seen performing standard airway maneuvers including removal of foreign bodies, lifting the chin or moving the jaw to move the tongue forward. The nurse also prevents shock by way of managing the circulatory system. This is done by controlling bleeding, or giving blood transfusions to replace significant blood loss.

Completing immediate care of an RTA patient to the emergency room unit is exposure of the patient's body. This is done by removing or cutting off the patient's clothes to enable effective visual examination of the entire body. It is during this examination that the extent of lacerations, cuts and injuries are identified and managed. Also, as patients could be at risk of a drop in body temperature, the vital signs (which include the checking of temperature, blood pressure and respiration) is done at this moment. The nurse, after doing these assessments, may decide, based on clinical findings, on which member of the health team should urgently continue with the care of the patient. A study at the Accident Centre of a tertiary hospital in Ghana noted the importance of 'good clinical decision making' during the process of emergency and routine care of accident patients (Ohene, 2008). Some of the issues that put nurses in dilemma, particularly when there are few nurses to take these decisions of triage, include 'who needs the most urgent care?'; 'who should go to the theatre first?' and 'who needs intensive care management?' It was reported that most often, nurses' decisions on clinical issues are right. It was however not stated how good decisions made by nurses are measured, but it was noted that they often use patient outcome to measure the decisions they take. Patient outcome is one of the accepted methods of measuring good or bad clinical decision but not the ultimate (Baron, 2004)

Routine Care of RTA Patient in Hospital Setting

After being satisfied with the primary survey assessment, the nurse continues to provide comfort, relieves patients' pain and puts broken parts in good alignment for immobilization of the part(s) involved. The nurse then calls the doctor who comes to continue with the care. However, in fatal accidents which involve large numbers of passengers, doctors do not wait to be called; instead, they come out and assist with care as soon as the cases arrive at reception (Ohene, 2008).

This stage of care, often referred to as the secondary survey, also focuses on systematic and thorough assessment of the patient from head to toe and front to back. By the end of this stage, all injuries should be identified, either as confirmed or as yet to be ruled out (Hardy & Barrett, 2003). The main goal of this stage is to reduce the incidence of delayed diagnosis or missed diagnosis. The assessment and diagnostic findings direct the plan for definitive care. Usually, the plan may include discharging minor injury patient(s), transferring patient(s) from the ER unit to a higher level or specialty facility, or admitting them to the hospital. At this stage also, nurses recognize the importance of reassurance for patients who may require admission. They have found that the sudden nature of the accident, unfamiliarity of the emergency environment, lack of knowledge of the outcome of care, and general anxiety can cause complications in newly admitted patients (Hallgrimsdottir, 2001; Murphy & Nightingale, 2002; Redley, Beanland & Botti, 2003; Williams et al., 2000).

Surgery-related interventions are among the routine steps taken for RTI patients. The nurse sees to the booking of patients for theatre and the patients are pre-operatively prepared. Pre-operative preparation includes physical, psychological, physiological and spiritual preparations (Hardy, 2003; Leistra et al., 1999). The nurses ensure that the needed items for theatre are gathered. After theatre, some patients are brought back to the emergency room for post-operative care. Sometimes there are other patients who may not have been to the theatre but due to lack of beds in the main wards, they are nursed in the emergency unit until they recover and are discharged. Thus, nurses often have to give routine care in addition to the emergency services they render to patients (Kitson, 1999).

Complications and Challenges of Nursing RTA Patients

It has been noted that the presence of multiple injured patients presents great challenges to accident and emergency nursing staff (Koch & Taylor, 1996). Subsequently, the failure to recognize and treat traumatic injuries correctly and promptly tends to cause early morbidity and mortality (Hadfield–law, 2000). Meanwhile, disability following to road traffic injuries now ranks ninth among the causes of disability, but is projected to rise to third by 2020 for myriad reasons (Johnell and Kanis, 2004).

Following RTA injuries and management, it has been reported that adverse reactions to injury and disability may occur. It is also noted that the consequences and after-effects of road traffic accidents have been neglected or under-emphasized (Michaud, Murray & Bloom, 2001). However, few researchers in this area seem to have made significant findings. Among the complications commonly identified are pain, disproportionate disability and psychiatric complications. Thus, the consequences of road accidents for victims remain significant, even one year after the accident, with pain identified as the most frequently reported after-effect associated with the least severely injured cases. Other effects reported in the literature include post-traumatic stress disorder (PTSD), anxiety and travel anxiety. These are among the psychological symptoms that have been reported that have received less attention, along with fatigue, fluctuating moods and difficulty in concentration, as well as nightmares and impaired memory (Taylor & Koch, 1995).

Consequently, literature is also scarce on the management of these complications following RTAs. Among the few suggestions that have been found are contributions by Brom et al. (2006) who acknowledged that although counseling is appreciated by traffic victims, it could not be proved to be effective in preventing disorders. Bordow and Porritt (1979)also state that crisis intervention is effective in helping patients to function normally 3-4 months after injury and may reduce the length of hospitalization. In another study, Modaghegh, Roudsari and Sajadehchi (2002) reported that inadequate medical information about the injury and the prognosis, as well as a lack of psychosocial support is associated with a higher risk of complications. They therefore suggest that a holistic approach to the care of victims of RTA is important. It is their view that early intervention as a routine practice in medical care might enable the injured to cope better with the trauma of a traffic injury and to recover from the injury itself.

Areas needing Attention to Reduce RTAs and Improve Care for Accident Victims in Ghana

Our road system needs to see improvement to reduce RTAs and also promote easy transportation of accident victims to the hospitals.

All road users must be educated on road regulations in order to avoid accidents. Drivers in particular must be properly trained and licensed. The public should also be educated on first aid and other things to do to help accident victims in their communities.

A national policy and guidelines must be formulated as to how trauma victims should be cared for and this should take into consideration the essential trauma care protocols. There is the need to intensify public education on how to handle accident victims at accident scenes and on the way to health facilities. Non-formal institutions that take care of some accident victims such as herbal medical practitioners must be identified and their procedures supervised.

The national ambulance system must be empowered to work effectively. Health training schools should start training accident and emergency nurse specialists. There is the need to also start training nurse practitioners to help take care of minor injuries independently. All health facilities must create accident and emergency units across the country with at least one accident and emergency nurse assigned to manage the facility. There must be regular in-service training and continuous educative programmes in accident and emergency care.

To facilitate immediate care for accident victims, the National Health Insurance Scheme should cover all initial care required by accident victims within the period of hospitalization. There should be enough equipment in all accident and emergency units. Emergency staff must be adequately remunerated. Some form of debriefing and continuous counseling must be initiated and made available to nursing staff as this helps them deal with their emotions after the death of patients at the accident centre, and prepares and strengthens them to get back to work in a stable emotional state.

Conclusion

Nursing management of RTA patients is not an event but a process which involves various steps and the challenges accompanying them. Training and acquisition of skills is essential in giving trauma care. It is time for policy makers to expand specialist training of emergency nurses to all the 10 regions and also include other health workers in the field of accident and emergency care in Ghana. Adequate acquisition of skills and fair distribution of skilled teams across the country will contribute to the decrease in deaths caused by road traffic accidents.

References

Aidoo, E.N., Amoh-Gyimah, R., & Ackaah, W. (2013). The effect of road and environmental characteristics on pedestrian hit and run accidents in Ghana. *Accident Analysis and Prevention*, 53, 23-27.

Afukaar, F. K., Antwi, P. & Ofosu-Amaah, S. (2003). Pattern of road traffic injuries in Ghana: implications for control. *Injury Control and Safety Promotion*, 10(1-2), 69–76.

Ghana National Road Safety Campaign. (2010). Annual Report 2010. Available from: http://www.nrsc.gov.gh/ assets/2010%20annual%20 report.pdf.

Baron, J. (2004). Normative models of judgment and decision making. *Blackwell Handbook of Judgment and Decision Making. London: Blackwell*, 19–36.

Bordow, S. & Porritt, D. (1979). An experimental evaluation of crisis intervention. *Social Science & Medicine. Part A: Medical Psychology & Medical Sociology*, 13, 251–256.

Brennan, P. (2002). Accident and emergency: theory into practice. *Emergency Medicine Journal: EMJ*, 19(1), 93.

Cornwell III, E. E. et al. (2000). Emergency medical services (EMS) vs non-EMS transport of critically injured patients: a prospective evaluation. *Archives of Surgery*, 135(3), 315.

Curtis, K., Murphy, M., Hoy, S. & Lewis, M. J. (2009). The emergency nursing assessment process—A structured framework for a systematic approach. *Australasian Emergency Nursing Journal*, 12(4), 130–136.

Damsere-Derry, J., Ebel, B.E., Mock, C.N., Afukaar, F., & Donkor, P. (2010) Pedestrian's injury patterns in Ghana. Accident Analysis and Prevention 42(4), 1080-1088.

Daniels, R. J., & Fulcher, R. A. (1997). An unusual cause of rib fracture following a road traffic accident. *Journal of Accident & Emergency Medicine*, 14(2), 113–114.

Dolan, B., & Holt, L. eds. (2007). *Accident & emergency: theory into practice.* London: Baillière Tindall. Available at: http://books.google.com.gh

Dunn, M. J. G., Gwinnutt, C. L., & Gray, A. J. (2007). Critical care in the emergency department: patient transfer. *Emergency Medicine Journal*, 24(1), 40–44.

Hallgrimsdottir, E. M. (2001). Accident and emergency nurses' perceptions and experiences of caring for families. *Journal of clinical nursing*, 9(4), 611–619.

Hardy, M., & Barrett, C. (2003). Interpreting trauma radiographs. *Journal of Advanced Nursing*, 44(1), 81–87.

Ingram, L. (1995). Roy's adaptation model and accidentand emergency nursing. *Accident and Emergency Nursing*, 3(3), 150–153. doi:10.1016/S0965-2302(95)80010-7

Jacobs, G., Aeron-Thomas, A., Astrop, A., & Britain, G. (2000). *Estimating global road fatalities.* Crowthorne: Transport Research Laboratory.

Jacoby, S. F., Ackerson, T. H., & Richmond, T. S. (2006). Outcome from serious injury in older adults. *Journal of Nursing Scholarship*, 38(2), 133–140.

Johnell, O., & Kanis, J. A. (2004). An estimate of the worldwide prevalence, mortality and disability associated with hip fracture. *Osteoporosis International*, 15(11), 897–902.

Koch, W. J., & Taylor, S. (1996). Assessment and treatment of motor vehicle accident victims. *Cognitive and Behavioral Practice*, 2(2), 327–342.

Kopits, E., & Cropper, M. (2005). Traffic fatalities and economic growth. *Accident Analysis & Prevention*, 37(1), 169–178.

Lagarde, E. (2007). Road traffic injury is an escalating burden in Africa and deserves proportionate research efforts. *PLOS Medicine*, 4(6), 170.

Liberman, M., Branas, C., Mulder, D. S., Lavoie, A., & Sampalis, J. S. (2004). Advanced Versus Basic Life Support in the Pre-Hospital Setting -- The Controversy between the 'Scoop and Run' and the 'Stay and Play' Approach to the Care of the Injured Patient. *International Journal of Disaster Medicine*, 2(1-2), 9–17.

MacFarlane, C., & Benn, C. A. (2003). Evaluation of emergency medical services systems: a classification to assist in determination of indicators. *Emergency Medicine Journal, 20*(2), 188–191.

Mayou, R., & Bryant, B. (2003). Consequences of road traffic accidents for different types of road user. *Injury, 34*(3), 197–202.

Mayou, Richard, & Bryant, B. (2001). Outcome in consecutive emergency department attenders following a road traffic accident. *The British Journal of Psychiatry, 179*(6), 528–534.

McConnell, J., Eyres, R., & Nightingale, J. (2008). The Skull and Face. *Interpreting Trauma Radiographs,* 262–277.

Mckay, H. (2006). Trauma Nurse Practitioners-Baptism by fire! Variations in role orientation. *Journal of Trauma Nursing, 13*(3), 102–104.

Michaud, C. M., Murray, C. J. L., & Bloom, B. R. (2001). Burden of disease— implications for future research. *JAMA: the Journal of the American Medical Association, 285*(5), 535–539.

Mock, C., Arreola-Risa, C., & Quansah, R. (2003). Strengthening care for injured persons in less developed countries: a case study of Ghana and Mexico. *Injury Control and Safety Promotion, 10*(1-2), 45–51.

Mock, C. N., Jurkovich, G. J., Arreola-Risa, C., Maier, R. V., others. (1998). Trauma mortality patterns in three nations at different economic levels: implications for global trauma system development. *The Journal of Trauma and Acute Care Surgery, 44*(5), 804–814.

Mock, Charles, Kobusingye, O., Anh, L. V., Afukaar, F., & Arreola-Risa, C. (2005). Human resources for the control of road traffic injury. *Bulletin of the World Health Organization, 83*(4), 294–300.

Modaghegh, M. H. S., Roudsari, B. S. & Sajadehchi, A. (2002). Prehospital trauma care in Tehran: Potential Areas for Improvement. *Prehospital Emergency Care, 6*(2), 218–223.

Murphy, F., & Nightingale, A. (2002). Accident and emergency nurses as researchers: exploring some of the ethical issues when researching sensitive topics. *Accident and Emergency Nursing, 10*(2), 72–77.

Murray, C. J. L., Lopez, A. D., & others. (1997). Alternative projections of mortality and disability by cause 1990-2020: Global Burden of Disease Study. *Lancet, 349*(9064), 1498–1504.

Naci, H., Chisholm, D., & Baker, T. D. (2009). Distribution of road traffic deaths by road user group: a global comparison. *Injury Prevention, 15*(1), 55–59.

Nantulya, V. M., & Reich, M. R. (2002a). The neglected epidemic: road traffic injuries in developing countries. *British Medical Journal, 324*(7346), 1139.

Nantulya, V. M., & Reich, M. R. (2002b). The neglected epidemic: road traffic injuries in developing countries. *British Medical Journal, 324*(7346), 1139.

Nirula, R., Talmor, D., & Brasel, K. (2005). Predicting significant torso trauma. *The Journal of Trauma and Acute Care Surgery, 59*(1), 132–135.

Nyström, M. (2002). Inadequate Nursing Care in an Emergency Care Unit in Sweden: Lack of a Holistic Perspective. *Journal of Holistic Nursing, 20*(4), 403–417.

Ohene, L.A. (2008). *Nursing management of road traffic accident victims.* University of Ghana, *Unpublished MPhil Thesis.*

Olive, P. (2003). The holistic nursing care of patients with minor injuries attending the A&E department. *Accident and Emergency Nursing, 11*(1), 27–32. doi:10.1016/S0965-2302(02)00130-3

Osei-Ampofo, M., Oduro, G., Oteng, R., Zakariah, A., Jacquet, G., & Donkor, P. (2013). The evolution and current state of emergency care in Ghana. *African Journal of Emergency Medicine, 3*(2), 52–58. doi:10.1016/j.afjem.2012.11.006.

Ozgediz, D., Hsia, R., Weiser, T., Gosselin, R., Spiegel, D., Bickler, S., Dunbar, P. & McQueen, K. (2009a). Population health metrics for surgery: effective coverage of surgical services in low-income and middle-income countries. *World Journal of Surgery, 33*(1), 1–5.

Ozgediz, D., Hsia, R., Weiser, T., Gosselin, R., Spiegel, D., Bickler, S., Dunbar, P. & McQueen, K. (2009b). Population health metrics for surgery: effective coverage of surgical services in low-income and middle-income countries. *World Journal of Surgery, 33*(1), 1–5.

Parry, N. G., & Girotti, M. J. (2008). Assessment of physical injury, acute pain and disability consequent to motor vehicle collision. *Motor vehicle collisions: Medical, psychosocial, and legal consequences,* 49–60.

Razzak, J. A., & Kellermann, A. L. (2002). Emergency medical care in developing countries: is it worthwhile? *Bulletin of the World Health Organization, 80*(11), 900–905.

Redley, B., Beanland, C., & Botti, M. (2003). Accompanying critically ill relatives in emergency departments. *Journal of Advanced Nursing, 44*(1), 88–98.

Sampalis, J. S., Tamim, H., Denis, R., Boukas, S., Ruest, S. A., Nikolis, A., & others. (1997). Ineffectiveness of on-site intravenous lines: is prehospital time the culprit? *The Journal of Trauma*, 43(4), 608.

Sauaia, A., Moore, F. A., Moore, E. E., Moser, K. S., Brennan, R., Read, R. A., & Pons, P. T. (1995). Epidemiology of trauma deaths: a reassessment. *The Journal of Trauma and Acute Care Surgery*, 38(2), 185–193.

Taylor, S., & Koch, W. J. (1995). Anxiety disorders due to motor vehicle accidents: Nature and treatment. *Clinical Psychology Review*, 15(8), 721–738. World Health Organisation. Deaths and DALY estimates for 2002 by cause for WHO Member States. World Health Organisation. Available from: http://www.who.int/entity/healthinfo/statisticsbodg deathdalyestimates.xls.

Chapter Six
A historical description of the emergence of HIV/AIDS in Ghana
Prudence P. Mwini-Nyaledzigbor

Introduction

The HIV/AIDS epidemic has been the subject of many interventions since the first cases were reported in the early 1980s around the world and in Ghana in 1986. The US Centers for Disease Control (CDC) and ministries of health (MOH) of various countries in the world have been monitoring and following the spread of the disease. In Ghana, the Ministry of Health (MOH) HIV Sentinel Surveillance System (HSSS) has been monitoring and following the trend of spread of the disease (Ministry of Health, 2001) and the various care and management interventions. This chapter will discuss the historical trends of the HIV/AIDS epidemic in Ghana and the emerging issues in the nursing care, preventive strategies, treatment and management of people living with HIV/AIDS in Ghana to date.

The Inception of HIV/AIDS in the World

The Acquired Immune Deficiency Syndrome (AIDS) epidemic is a serious health and development problem in many countries. The number of infected persons increased rapidly after 1981 when the first AIDS-related cases were reported by the Centers for Diseases Control (CDC) in the United States (CDC, 1989). The Joint United Nations Programme on AIDS (UNAIDS, 2000) estimated in 2000 that the number of adults and children living with AIDS worldwide was 36.1 million. Of these, 25.3 million were in sub-Saharan Africa. UNAIDS (2000) also reported that 3.0 million people had already died from the disease by 2000. The estimated number of children orphaned by AIDS in that year was 13.2 million, with 12.1 million of these in Africa. The estimated number of children who were newly infected with HIV globally in 2000 was 600,000, with 520,000 of these children living in sub-Saharan Africa (UNAIDS, 2000).

Historical Perspectives on HIV/AIDS in Ghana

AIDS in Ghana has had a short but devastating history in the 26 years since the first AIDS cases were reported in March 1986 (Ministry of Health, 2001). This writer observed that it all started as a rumour. Then the Ministry of Health found that it was dealing with a disease. As the years went by, we all realized that it was an epidemic, and then everyone knew that a tragedy was occurring.

In the early years of the epidemic, approximately 3 percent of the adult population was infected (Ministry of Health, 2001). In 1986 the prevalence rate was 2.9 percent; it dropped to 2.6 percent in 1999 and then rose to 3.6 percent in 2001 and 3.4 percent in 2004 and later to 3.6 percent in the same year. In 1999, HIV prevalence among sex workers in Accra was 78.5 percent and 82 percent in Kumasi, respectively (GAC, 2004). The Ministry of Health had already initiated the HIV Sentinel Surveillance System in 1992 to monitor the trends of spread of the disease in the general population. The HIV Sentinel Survey report plus other data provide the primary data for estimation and projection of the impact of HIV/AIDS in Ghana.

Once HIV became established, rapid transmission rates in the urban centres made the epidemic far more devastating than in the rural settings (Ministry of Health, 2001). The accelerated spread in the urban centres was due to a combination of widespread rural-urban migration, high ratio of women in the urban population, the low status of women, and the prevalence of sexually transmitted infections. It was initially thought that sex workers played a large part in the accelerated transmission rate in Ghana. This was later proven to be false as the HIV transmission was found to be significantly present among the general population of various occupations and marital status. The number of HIV positive persons was estimated to be between 400,000 and 600,000 with an infection rate of 200 persons per day. Individuals between the ages 15 and 49 years were the most affected (Ministry of Health, 2001). Among women, the highest prevalence of AIDS cases occurred in the 25-29 years age group whereas among men the highest prevalence was in the 35-39 years age group.

The Health Sentinel Surveillance System of the National AIDS Control Programme and Sexually Transmitted Infections (NACP/STI) of the Health Ministry (2001) then began to make projections of the infection rates in order to plan preventive programmes. Between 1994 and 2000 the MOH sponsored a yearly surveillance of all sites in the country. An analysis of the surveillance data indicated that HIV prevalence among the 15-49 year olds rose from 2.7 percent in 1994 to 3.0 percent in 2000. There was certainly a danger that HIV prevalence in Ghana could increase in the future in the absence of preventive interventions and strategic care and management plans at a time when there was a lack of concrete evidence on the real causes of HIV/AIDS.

Again, the projections of HIV prevalence in the age group 15 - 49 were for an increase from 3 percent in 2000 to 4.7 percent by 2004 and 9 percent in 2014. The projections, therefore, meant that there were going to be 72,000 HIV-positive individuals by 2004. The report also indicated that the number of HIV infections would continue to rise to more than a million by 2014 (Ministry of Health, 2001) and families and communities would be greatly affected. From 1986 to 2000, the cumulative number of AIDS deaths was estimated at 160,000. This was an indication of the seriousness of the epidemic in Ghana. It meant additional responsibilities and an extra burden for the extended family to cater for AIDS patients and their dependents.

Heterosexual contact and mother-to-child transmission constituted the two major routes of HIV transmission in Ghana. Transmission through heterosexual contact formed 80 percent and mother-to-child transmission constituted 15 percent. Transmission through contaminated needles, blood and blood products and other routes constituted the remaining 5 percent (Ministry of Health, 2001). The 'other' mode of transmission was thought to include the use of skin piercing instruments including knives, blades, and thorns used by untrained traditional healers for scarification and application of herbal preparations, female genital mutilation (FGM) and circumcision by untrained circumcisers popularly known as *wanzam* (Ministry of Health, 2001). Barbers, hairdressers, poor handling of body fluids and the acceptance of injections from "quack doctors" was also a suspected route of HIV infection transmission in Ghana in the early days. Even insects such as mosquitoes, handshakes or the use of communal drinking cups were all suspected routes for transmission until the Centers for Disease Control and Prevention ([CDC], 1999) Guidelines were published and clarified the actual modes for transmission of HIV.

After more than three decades, one critically assess and conceptualize the evolution of AIDS as three successive epidemics (Herek & Glunt, 1988). The first epidemic (Herek & Glunt, 1988) remained hidden and represented people who were infected with the virus. It has been estimated that, the median HIV prevalence for 2009 was 2.9 percent while that for 2010 was 2.0 percent and 2011 was 2.1 percent respectively. HIV prevalence in urban areas was higher than in rural areas, with the mean and median HIV prevalence of urban communities were 3.5 percent and 3.6 percent compared to 2.4 percent and 2.2 percent in rural areas respectively. The highest prevalence was recorded within the age group 40-44 years (4.0 percent) and the lowest (1.9 percent) in the 15-19 year age group. The urban centres accounted for higher rates due to work force mobility from original settlements, resulting in prolonged separation from spouses left behind and freedom from the cultural, societal and community watch.

The prevalence of HIV among the 15-24 year age group, whose prevalence is usually used as a proxy for new HIV infections in the country, saw an increase from 1.9 percent in 2008 to 2.1 percent in 2009, according to the National AIDS Control Programme/Sexually Transmission Infections (NACP/STI, 2009). HIV annual projections and prevalence in the general population were based on HIV Sentinel Survey (HSS) data compiled as an annual, cross-sectional survey conducted by the NACP/STI in 40 selected urban and rural antenatal settings across Ghana. Other ways of monitoring HIV infections included health care provider counseling and testing, and HIV voluntary counseling and testing. Kyei-Boateng (2012) reported on adolescent HIV increases, with 40 percent of adolescents in some junior high schools (JHS) and 40 percent in some senior high schools (SHS) as well as 20 percent at tertiary institutions found to be HIV-positive. Schools, colleges and universities provide wider exposure for adolescents and young adults to unsupervised peer influence and numerous temptations. There is, therefore, the need for intensified health education messages in educational institutions on prevention of HIV/AIDS infection and the provision of better school health services.

The second AIDS epidemic (Herek & Glunt, 1988) is mainly visible and includes those with the symptoms of AIDS. In 2008, national estimates and projections for HIV-positive population in 2009 amounted to 240, 802. The people with HIV/AIDS comprised 219,600 adults and 21,202 children, with an annual AIDS death toll of 17,058 (NACP/STI, 2009). Trends in HIV transmission rose among adolescents due to conservative cultural beliefs that prohibit sex education for young people.

There is stigma attached to HIV/AIDS in Ghana which has fuelled the third epidemic described by Herek and Glunt (1988). According to other researchers too, (Mill, 2003; Mwinituo & Mill, 2006; Wright and Mwini-Nyaledzigbor, 2010) stigma is itself an epidemic and it is social in nature, leading to secrecy. This third epidemic consisting of self-stigmatisation and social stigma is often hidden, sometimes visible but is always present (Herek & Glunt, 1988). Knowledge of the effects of AIDS-related stigma is important. Stigma tends to have an impact on the preparedness of individuals to disclose and subsequently seek care, treatment and support. So in Ghana, although HIV prevalence is low, it is firmly established across the whole society, and there are sub-populations with higher prevalence and risk of transmission that remain as the reservoir for sustaining the epidemic. Thus, HIV/AIDS has become a chronic condition that requires both institutional and community-based approaches to its prevention, care and management.

Worldview of Ghanaians on HIV/AIDS: Scenes of Confusion, Stigma and Despondency

HIV infection and transmission in Ghana has been 'shrouded in secrecy' (Mill, 2003 pg.6). In the mid 1980s and early1990s, the HIV/AIDS epidemic was characterized as a period of confusion, gossip and rumour as to the nature of AIDS and its causes in many Ghanaian communities. The cause of AIDS was still unclear in the early 1980s although it was thought to be an infectious agent, and probably a virus (Marx, 1983). Very little was known about transmission and public anxiety and fears were high. Everybody (including health care professionals) was simply bewildered. With many questions unanswered, there were numerous misconceptions, with people thinking that one can get HIV through a handshake or sitting on a chair used by a person with AIDS or stepping over the urine voided by an AIDS patient (Mwini-Nyaledzigbor & Wright, 2011). It was even said that 'HIV can be transmitted just by chance through touching the big toe of an AIDS person'. Additionally, confusion with other diseases such as malaria led to over-estimation of the transmissibility of HIV and added to the fear surrounding the virus.

Fear quickly bred stigma attached to people infected with HIV. Stigma was often related to the association of HIV with prostitution, promiscuity, 'basabasa' and other high-risk lifestyle behaviour (Anarfi, 1995; Mill, 2003 pg. 8). As the current writer observed, in the early days, HIV was a disease for prostitutes. For example, a woman in a miniskirt or one that appeared slim were the ones supposed to have AIDS. People with HIV were often not aware that they had the disease until they had progressed to the final stages when death was often imminent in the then absence of ART. This fact, coupled with the lack of any effective opportunistic infection preventive treatment, meant that the diagnosis of HIV was equated to the issuance of a death sentence. This led to great reluctance by Ghanaians to be tested for the virus. "Why get tested if there is no treatment and no cure; if you were sent home to die; shunned by your family and neighbours; I'll rather take poison and die; all die be die; I prefer to die with my flesh than to grow lean like a stick and die" (Mill, 2003; Wright & Mwinituo, 2010, pg. 39).

AIDS and Stigma in Ghana

According to Goffman (1963), stigma is a term used in Classical Greece to mean a bodily sign cut or burnt into a person, thus denoting, for example, criminals whose moral character was considered tarnished. Goffman (1963) also indicated that stigma expresses the perceptual meanings or mental images through which a person is viewed as inferior, dirty and contagious to others. The stigma thus labels the person as untouchable, abnormal or morally spoiled or weak and to be avoided by individuals, for various reasons and on traditional stance in a variety of context within any given society. The stigmatized, being aware of the "mark", in turn tries in everyday life to avoid any social contact, even with people they know, leading to isolation and self-stigmatization.

AIDS as an illness has attributes that makes it likely to evoke stigma. Various interpretations have been given to the sexual nature of HIV infection and transmission by individuals and groups in society. Given their strong cultural and religious beliefs, it is not surprising that some Ghanaians proclaimed that AIDS is a punishment from God for sins committed. Stigma and discrimination worsen the plight of HIV-positive persons and this calls for effective interventions to reduce the psychosocial and economic burden of AIDS.

Again, stigma serves as a huge barrier to disclosure of HIV status (Wright & Mwinituo, 2010). The impact of being diagnosed with HIV on the social lives and economic activities of the affected individual was the driving force for the persistent refusal of most people to disclose their HIV-positive status. Other reasons usually include negative emotional experiences; quality of life versus longing to die without disclosure and continued social participation in economic survival activities. The psychosocial experiences of a person diagnosed with HIV/AIDS stems from the way society will view that fellow. The stigma and discrimination often result in HIV-positive persons developing various negative feelings including fear, sense of loss, grief, anger, guilt, denial and low self-esteem (van Dyk, 2008; Wright & Mwinituo, 2010). These negative feelings can lead to suicidal ideations, social isolation and depression.

There is also a type of stigma known as associative stigma or "courtesy stigma" (Goffman, 1963) which is extended to people who are connected either by blood relationship or affine or friendship to the person being stigmatized. Examples of such connectedness include informal caregivers, children, family, and others. The stigmatized person and the associates are likely to react with secrecy, denial or defensiveness and may suffer depression.

Examples of Associative Stigma

In the early days of HIV/AIDS, associative stigma was predominant as families battled alone with their relatives who contracted HIV and developed AIDS. Mwinituo and Mill (2006) described associative stigma as a huge prison-like wall surrounding both the caregiver and the HIV/AIDS patient, keeping the two in isolation. This led to despair and desperation on the part of the patient and the caregiver. The world beyond the wall of stigma was hostile, frightening and uncaring. Doctors, nurses and other healthcare professionals were part of this world beyond the wall because they also stigmatized and discriminated against the "inmates" within the wall by remaining silent, not caring for the patient appropriately, and ignoring the caregiver.

The caregivers felt as if they were no longer part of this world. They verbalized this in various ways. The observation of one of the participants in the study, illustrates the feeling of informal caregivers: *"Sometimes when I want to go out and buy things, I feel shy. The moment I meet people I know I feel shy of myself. Because my husband has AIDS, I feel people know I also have AIDS. No words! Those who know me simply stare at me and I quickly get the message and disappear".*

The associative stigma also forced caregivers to provide care to their relatives in absolute secrecy. This situation put a lot of strain on caregivers because while caring responsibilities were difficult, great efforts were also put into 'hiding' the patient and all caring activities thereby created a major burden for caregivers. One participant indicates: *"….So, for fear of the fact that people will get to know that it is AIDS, I usually hide to do the laundry, and sneak out to dry them at dawn and go away before the other tenants could wake up to see me."*

However, the absence of social sanctions and ability to speak out against AIDS-related stigma and discrimination continues to fuel the flames of stigma. This is particularly so because there are no sanctions against stigmatization and discrimination against people living with HIV and AIDS. The lack of sanctions and avenues for social support systems is embodied in these statements made by some HIV/AIDS patients studied: *"as AIDS patients, we have no access to legal aid services; besides, no law works in Ghana here; no privacy and confidentiality in the court rooms".* The lack of trust in law enforcement agencies to enforce the rights of HIV and AIDS persons in the country and to shield them from further public exposure and ridicule was the concern of all the participants in that study.

Ghana's Response to the HIV/AIDS Epidemic

The health sector has been the vital and lead technical partner in the country's response to HIV and AIDS. The Ghana Health Service (GHS) and the National AIDS/STI Control Programme (NACP/STI) of the Ministry of Health provide prevention, treatment, care and support services as well as vital information for action. As stated above, the mid-1980s period was characterised by inadequate knowledge of and insufficient response to HIV and AIDS in Ghana .

In the absence of treatment or cure for HIV/AIDS, government strategies had to focus on prevention. The prevention efforts have focused on encouraging people to revise their sexual behaviour by abstaining from sex, being faithful to one partner or having fewer partners, or using condoms consistently and correctly. For adolescents particularly, the message has been to delay first sex. However, prevention efforts in Ghana were often confronted with opposition from some religious authorities. The Christian leaders found prevention campaigns such as condom promotion difficult to reconcile with their faith and instead recommended total abstinence as a better option. This seems to be not realistic, considering the instinctual nature of human sexuality.

Coming into the new millennium, Ghana's response to the HIV/AIDS epidemic has benefited considerably from a continued and favourable policy environment, reflected in the formulation of supportive policies and guidelines, strong advocacy and resource mobilization. Soon after the establishment of the Ghana AIDS Commission by an Act of Parliament in December 2001, decentralized institutional structures for policy implementation, coordination and management were created (GAC, 2004). There is also widespread civil society participation. Other stakeholders include governmental and non-governmental organizations, faith-based organizations and community-based sub-projects decentralised to the District Assemblies (Ghana AIDS Commission, 2004).

The national response considered the epidemic not only as a disease to be treated with bio-medical methods but also to be seen as a developmental and human rights issue (Ghana AIDS Commission, 2004; NACP/STI and MOH, 2001). The Ghana AIDS Commission adopted a holistic, coordinated and multisectoral approach through HIV/AIDS policy formulation, resource mobilization, coordination and supervision as well as the involvement of civil society in a strategic management plan (Ghana AIDS Commission, 2004).

A national strategic framework was developed with the objective of reducing the prevalence rates among the 15-49 year old group by 30 percent, create an enabling environment for people living with HIV and AIDS, improve service delivery and mitigate the social impact of HIV and AIDS on families and individuals in communities. In addition, the aim was to establish an institutional framework for the co-ordination and implementation of HIV and AIDS programmes in the country (Ghana AIDS Commission, 2004).

The intervention areas of the national response focused on awareness creation, prevention of mother-to-child transmission of HIV, provision of the needed support and care for people living with HIV and AIDS (PLWHA), treatment, research, HIV Counseling and Testing (HCT), periodic screening for opportunistic infections (OIs) in PLWHA, and monitoring and evaluation of all HIV and AIDS activities within the country (Ghana AIDS Commission, 2004; NACP/STI, 2007).

Priority intervention areas were the prevention of new infections through safer sex particularly with the use of condoms, management of sexually transmitted infections, blood screening for safety, infection control in the care of patients and prevention of mother-to-child transmission of HIV (Ghana AIDS Commission, 2004; NACP/STI, 2007).

The Arrival of Antiretroviral Therapy in Ghana

`Treatment and support of persons living with HIV and AIDS in Ghana started in mid-2003 and critical reviews were made to include a change in the viral load (CD4) count criteria from <250 to <350 cells /mm3 for ART eligibility as well as clear listing of antiretroviral drugs for use in Ghana. Guidelines for ART (NACP/STI, 2009) were immediately put together according to the World Health Organization's (WHO) specifications.

Ghana made several gains through the utilization of a Global Fund disbursement for HIV/AIDS, tuberculosis and malaria, worth US$4.9 million in 2004. The achievements made through a scale-up plan targeted for 2006 consisted of the organization and training of healthcare professionals, mostly public health nurses and nurse midwives who doubled as health educators, HIV/AIDS counselors and prescribers for prevention and treatment of opportunistic infections. Nurses facilitated in workshops as trainers of trainees and also contributed to the care and management of HIV/AIDS in several ways including HIV counseling and testing, prevention of mother-to-child transmission of HIV (PMTCT), training of traditional circumcisers (Kwanzaas) and traditional herbalists on HIV infection prevention, adherence counseling for PLWAs put on antiretroviral treatment (ART) and providing continuity of care to AIDS patients in their homes through home visiting. Nurses all over Ghana played pivotal roles in the care and management of HIV/AIDS clients in the following ways:

- HIV Counseling and Testing in all the three teaching hospitals and all regional and district hospitals.
- Prevention of mother-to-child transmission of HIV sites in all regional and district hospitals through screening and treatment of pregnant women.
- Management of opportunistic infections made available in all regional and district hospitals.
- Access to ART made available in all the three teaching hospitals, and all regional, and district hospitals.
- Supervision and distribution of nutritional supplements and food aid to PLWAs.

Funding of non-governmental organizations involved in HIV and AIDS activities was the prerogative function of the Ghana AIDS Commission (Ghana AIDS Commission, 2004; NACP/STI, 2007). The Commission's plans and achievements through the period from 2006 to 2012 and beyond included the establishment of antiretroviral therapy (ART) centers in all regional and district hospitals that are managed by nurses and doctors. Thus, care and management consisted of :

- universal access to care and support in regional and district hospitals;
- decentralization of national response in District Assemblies; and
- District Assemblies to take charge of monitoring and evaluation of HIV and AIDS activities (Ghana AIDS Commission, 2007).

Home-Based Care and Management of HIV/AIDS Patients in the mid-1980s

From the mid-1980s and through the 1990s, civil society, especially the family, played a vital role by providing home-based care for people with HIV and AIDS. This consisted of physical care as well as psycho-social and emotional support. In several cases, family members also consulted spiritual at some point in time in view of the AIDS patient's deteriorating condition.

Home-based care is the care given in the AIDS patient's home or place of abode. This care is usually given by a family member or a friend, usually referred to as the primary caregiver. In ideal circum-stances, the family caregiver is a blood relation who is designated to meet the specific needs of the AIDS patient. Many studies show that family caregivers for AIDS patients were their blood relations (Anarfi, 1995; Buning, 1996; Mwinituo and Anarfi, 2005) as a result of the huge stigma attached to AIDS that time. Thus the caregivers were mothers caring for their sick daughters, daughters and sons caring for their sick mothers, wives caring for their husbands and in some cases boyfriends caring for their fiancées. An 80-year old Madam Akwele (pseudonym) caring for her daughter put it this way:

> There is nobody, she is my daughter, and it is my duty
> to give care. The way the disease is, it takes only a
> blood relation to give care to afflicted persons.

The home-based care was often the best way to look after someone with AIDS as good basic care can be successfully provided in the home; people who are very sick and dying, often prefer to stay at home in their familiar surroundings especially when they know they cannot be cured in hospital. Furthermore, home-based care promotes a holistic approach to care. The physical, social, psychological, emotional, religious and spiritual needs of the patient can all be fulfilled by the family. However, home-based care also has certain potential problems for the family caregiver and the patient. Non-compliance with treatment often occurs as the patient or family caregiver does not know how or when to administer medications. Also, a lack of knowledge about the disease often hampers home-based care. The entire care giving can be very burdensome, despite the commitment of all the caregivers (Mwinituo, & Mill, 2006). Consequently, there were expressions of exhaustion, worry, fear and despair that constituted a heavy burden. Madam Aku, a mother caring for her daughter indicated:

> Now I am tired! I have been trying all I can but her sickness is getting worse and worse. I am now really tired. If she will go to toilet, she calls me, if she is to urinate, she calls me, and then I will lift her up onto a chamber pot.

Institutional (Hospital) Care of the AIDS Patient in the 1980s and 1990s

Before the advent of antiretroviral treatment (ART), care of the HIV-infected patient was focused on prophylaxis against opportunistic infections (OIs), management of OIs, ongoing prevention and end-of-life care in the nations' hospitals and clinics. An understanding of HIV, its transmission, and how it affects the body's immune system was important for nurses in their roles as clinicians, educators, patients' advocates and counselors. Nurses were given training through workshops about the new disease. AIDS patients were conveyed in and out of the hospitals to undergo rehydration or treatment for opportunistic infections.

The basic nursing care given to HIV and AIDS patients on admission often lasted for a few days or weeks and the patient was discharged to the family. Much as it is impossible to recommend any one care model for AIDS patients, the nursing process was the best guide to diagnosing problems and implementing care interventions for patients. Due to the large influx of patients and the heavy care demands placed by them, most nurses sooner or later developed symptoms of burnout, including physical exhaustion, fatigue, fear of vulnerability to HIV-infection, irritability, anger and strained relations with AIDS patients and their relatives (Laryea, 1993). Many family caregivers had no idea about infection prevention and could not afford detergents and antiseptic agents. Instead of some nurses teaching family caregivers how to make use of community resources to prevent infection in the home while providing care for AIDS patients, some nurses displayed negative attitudes to patients and their relatives.

Attitude of Health Care Professionals

Most terminal cases were cared for at homes and were only sent to the hospital when death was imminent. Family caregivers were never counseled. This resulted in the caregivers not knowing how to handle body discharges and protect themselves and other family members. It intensified the caregivers' fears about the disease. Caregivers could not recognize the terminal stages of AIDS while some nurses put aside their ethical principles and treated AIDS patients and their relatives unprofessionally and with disgust. The following statements from the study by Mwinituo and Mill (2006) depict the situation at the time:

A wife, caring for her husband and a child, pleaded with health professionals for respect:

> If we come to the hospital nurses should exercise patience with us, though we are having this disease we are still human beings. So far as we are not yet dead we are still human beings. They should respect us; the way they behave towards us is not fair so they should stop.

Another mother caring for her daughter on admission in the ward with AIDS could not hide her feelings about the attitude of nurses:

> When I send her to the hospital for admission they don't do anything for my daughter. They don't feed her, they don't clean her. One day, she fell from the bed and called the nurses; none of them bothered to help her

> *up. I went and saw her on the floor and I lifted her up.*
> *Some of the nurses are even rude to me and behave as*
> *if I am their rival.*

Patients and their relatives felt nurses and doctors were not treating them with respect. Above all, they called for recognition and respect, and pleaded with nurses to end the disregard meted out to HIV/AIDS persons and their family caregivers.

Currently, Ghana is among five West African countries that have seen HIV prevalence among young people decline by more than 25 percent between 2001 and 2010 (UNAIDS, 2010). There is access to ART and care services in all health institutions. It is now widely known and accepted that antiretroviral therapy (ART) can extend life expectancy, reduce viral load and lower the risk of HIV transmission. This has retarded the progress of HIV to AIDS and reversed greatly the influx of hospitals by AIDS patients thus bringing relief to nurses who provide care for AIDS patients.

Conclusion

This chapter has discussed the emergence of HIV and AIDS in Ghana and the responses to date. This has included Ghanaian society's views on HIV/AIDS in the 1980s and 1990s, AIDS stigma, and the advent of antiretroviral therapy. The paper has described the role played by the family in home-based care. It has also stressed the important role that nurses play in looking after HIV/AIDS patients on admission and in providing information and education on HIV/AIDS care for the benefit of home caregivers.

The issue of stigmatization remains a major constraint that works against proper care and management of the HIV/AIDS disease in Ghana. Although great progress has been made in Ghana since the inception of the disease, in particular, making available ART to PLWHA, the issue of stigma continues to discourage PLWHA from making their condition known and taking advantage of available treatment, particularly antiretroviral treatment (ART) which is now readily available in designated ART centres in Ghana's regional and district hospitals.

Negative attitudes of health professionals, including nurses, towards PLWHA also persist and education is required to reverse these negative attitudes which are born of misconceptions about transmission of the disease. HIV transmission and the ability to cope with its consequences cannot be isolated from the demographic, cultural, economic, social and political conditions of a country. Although Ghana has made great progress and achieved positive results in its response to the HIV/AIDS epidemic and AIDS-related deaths have fallen, health professionals, especially nurses, need to keep up the effort and should not relent in ensuring that PLWHA have access to available care and management.

References

Anarfi, J.K. (1995). The conditions and care of AIDS victims in Ghana: AIDS sufferers and their relatives. *Health Transition Review,* 5(Suppl.), 253-263.

Bunting, S. M. (1996). Persons with AIDS and their family caregivers: Negotiating the journey. *Journal of Family Nursing,* 2(4), 399-417.

Centres for Disease Control and Prevention. (1989; 1999; 2000). HIV and its transmission. Available at: http://www.cdcgov/hiv/resources/factsheets/. [Accessed 16 September 2012].

Ghana AIDS Commission (2004). National HIV/AIDS and sexually transmitted infection policy, 2004. Accra: Government Printing Office.

Goffman, E. (1963). Stigma: Notes on the management of spoiled identity. Englewood Cliffs: Prentice Hall.

Herek, G.M. & Glunt, E.K. (1988). An epidemic of stigma: Public reactions to AIDS. *Journal of American Psychologist,* 43(11), 886-891.

Kyei-Boateng, J. (2012, August 23). Adolescent HIV increases in Schools. *Daily Graphic.* p. 3.

Laryea, J.L. (1993). A Study of Knowledge and Attitudes of Ghanaian Nurses towards HIV/AIDS. Unpublished dissertation, University of Ghana.

Marx, J.L. (1983). 'Acquired Immune Deficiency Syndrome Abroad' Research News 2 December: 73. In: Kulsand, R. ed. (1986). AIDS: Papers from Science, 1982-1985. The American Association for the Advancement of Science.

Mill, J. E. (2003). Shrouded in secrecy: Breaking the news of HIV infection to Ghanaian women. *Journal of Transcultural Nursing,* 14(1), 6-16.

Ministry of Health (2001). Background, Projections on HIV/AIDS: Annual Report, 2001. Accra: Government Printing Office.

Mwinituo, P.P. & Anarfi, J.K. (2005). The Experiences of Informal Caregivers in the Management of AIDS Patients in Accra, Ghana. *Geographical Association*, 2, 82-88.

Mwinituo, P.P. & Mill, J. E. (2006). Stigma Associated with Ghanaian Caregivers of AIDS Patients. *Western Journal of Nursing Research*, 28(4), 369-390.

Mwinituo, P.P. & Wright, S.C.D. (2010). Lived Experiences of Ghanaian Women Diagnosed with HIV and AIDS. *African Journal of Nursing and Midwifery*, 12 (2), 36-47.

Mwini-Nyaledzigbor, P.P. and Wright, S.C.D. (2011). Misconceptions about HIV Infection Faced by Diagnosed Ghanaian Women. *African Journal of Midwifery and Women's Health*, 5(3),141-147.

National AIDS Control Programme/Sexually Transmitted Infection (2001). HIV sentinel survey report. Accra: Government Printing Office.

National AIDS Control Programme/Sexually Transmitted Infection (2007). HIV sentinel survey report. Accra: Government Printing Office.

National AIDS Control Programme/Sexually Transmitted Infection (2009). HIV sentinel survey report. Accra: Government Printing Office.

National AIDS Control Programme/Sexually Transmitted Infection Bulletin (2007). Accra: National AIDS Control Programme.

Increasing access to HIV treatment: the past, present and future. Publishers Quarterly Technical Bulletin Ghana: Government Printing Office.

United Nations Programme on HIV/AIDS (2000). Update report on global AIDS statistics. Available at: http://www.unaids update report hiv/aids/resources/factsheets/. [Accessed: 16 September 2012].

United Nations Programme on HIV/AIDS (2000). Overview report on the global HIV/AIDS epidemic. Available at: http://www.unaids update report hiv/aids/resources/factsheets/. [Accessed: 16 September 2012].

Van Dyk, A. (2008). *HIV/AIDS care and counseling: A multidisciplinary approach.* 3rd ed. South Africa: Pearson Education.

Chapter Seven
Implementation of the National Breastfeeding Policy in Ghana: Challenges and Future Prospects
Comfort K. Affram and *Ernestina S. Donkor*

Introduction

Breastfeeding is the natural and ideal way of feeding the infant. The appropriate feeding practices during these early stages of life are crucial for optimal development and child survival. It is believed that breast milk provides the child with an entire range of anti-infective substances and essential nutrients. This leads to prevention of malnutrition and its related illnesses, and consequently a decrease in child morbidity and mortality. The National Breastfeeding Policy was instituted to curb childhood malnutrition and decrease infant morbidity and mortality.

Malnutrition in infancy is a global problem with many fatal consequences. Children who have chronic malnutrition do not achieve their full growth potential (Grigsby, 2006). Malnutrition is associated with childhood killer diseases. A World Health Organization report on diseases that cause death among children less than five years old shows that these diseases are all associated with malnutrition (WHO, 2001a). Among other causes of deaths, 1.2 million children die annually in sub-Saharan Africa from acute respiratory infection, especially pneumonia, and from diarrhoea diseases (800,000), measles (500,000) and malaria (600,000).

The government of Ghana has been making efforts to tackle infant morbidity and mortality. One of its strategic plans is the promotion of exclusive breastfeeding. Under this strategic plan, it was recommended that children are breastfed exclusively from birth to six months before complementing breast milk with other food up to two years or more (Ghana Health Service, 2004). The purpose of this chapter is to describe the implementation of the National Breastfeeding Policy, highlight the challenges of its implementation and future prospects.

Breastfeeding Policy in Ghana

Based on the Millennium Development Goals, the Ghana of Government is committed to improving the health of the child (Ministry of Health, Ghana, 2006). The National Breastfeeding Policy states that "The Government/Ministry of Health shall seek to promote exclusive breastfeeding for about the first six (6) months of an infant's life and continuing breastfeeding with complementary feeds up to two (2) years or more..." (Ghana Health Service, 2003). Ghana passed a Breastfeeding Promotion Regulation 2000, L.I.1667 (Ghana Health Service, 2000) to support the policy. The focus of developing the National Breastfeeding Policy was to help decrease infant malnutrition and mortality in Ghana. There has been a slight decrease in IMR in the following years: 1988, 1993, 1998, 2003 and 2008 as 77, 66, 57, 64 and 50 per 1000 live births respectively (Ghana Statistical Service, 2008). In line with this policy, various strategies have been outlined in order to fulfill the desired goals. The strategies focus on breastfeeding education during the antenatal and postnatal periods. Other strategies centered on incorporation of the policy into curriculum and training programmes, and improving the conditions of working nursing mothers, and HIV infant feeding. One major strategy used to implement the breastfeeding policy in Ghana was the Baby-friendly Hospital Initiative training programme that was started in 1994. These included an 80-hour course for training of trainers in lactation management, an 18-hour course for maternity staff, and a breastfeeding course for hospital administrators and policy makers run by WHO/UNICEF and National Baby-Friendly Hospital Initiative assessors. Tutors and lecturers from nursing training institutions as well as doctors were trained in lactation management. Mother support group facilitators were also trained and in turn trained support groups in the communities, as stated in the Infant Baby Food Action Network Ghana Country Report (IBFAN, 2006).

Exclusive breastfeeding implies feeding the child with only breast milk (WHO, 2013). Thus breast milk substitutes, water, other liquids and solid foods are excluded. Exclusive breastfeeding for six months (compared to three to four months) has certain advantages. In addition to other benefits, it helps the mother to lose weight (Kramer & Kakuma, 2002). It also serves as an artificial family planning method by delaying ovulation. However, research has shown poorer iron status in infants who were exclusively breastfed for six months, as opposed to four months followed by partial breastfeeding to six months (WHO, 2001b). This evidence is likely to apply to populations where maternal iron status and infant endogenous stores are not optimal (WHO, 2001b). This implies that breastfeeding mothers must ensure that their diets contain sufficient iron.

In order to achieve a sustained reduction in child mortality and childhood malnutrition in Ghana, it is important for healthcare professionals to acquire significant knowledge of the policy and to put into into practice. The content of the policy must be widely disseminated. For example, mothers who are the implementers of the policy must be given the right information on breastfeeding to achieve the goals of the policy. When mothers are empowered with knowledge, malnutrition and morbidity problems in the child are more easily tackled. Studies have shown that health information and education significantly enhance mothers' knowledge of the importance of breastfeeding, initiation of lactation, frequency and other lactation practices. Maternal education is significant in feeding practices but higher educational level is not the key (Frost, Forste & Haas, 2004). Appoh and Krekling (2005) find that mothers' nutritional knowledge alone appears to be the crucial skill in improving children's nutritional status. They stated however, that such knowledge is acquired outside the classroom. The implication is that in communities where formal education is limited, it may be possible to impart nutritional knowledge with child nutrition educational programmes. Studies have shown improved nutritional level as a result of such programmes (Senbanjo, Adeodu & Adejuyige, 2007). Though malnutrition remains a crucial problem in Ghana, the policy has contributed to general awareness of the importance of exclusive breastfeeding.

Breastfeeding Practices in Relation to the Policy

Affram (2013) conducted a study entitled "Evidenced-Based Guidelines to Improve the Implementation of the National Breastfeeding Policy in Ghana" using mixed methods between 2009 and 2013. Ethical clearance was obtained from Ethical Review Committee of Noguchi Memorial Institute for Medical Research, University of Ghana. Three hundred mothers with their 400 children, 18 mother support groups and 35 midwives were recruited from Mamprobi community and polyclinic in Accra. The anthropometric measurements of the children were taken. It was found that mothers universally accepted exclusive breastfeeding as feeding the child only on breast milk for six months before giving other foods. However, the majority (83 percent) gave water to their children, especially bottled mineral water. The mothers did breastfeed their children but the majority was not practicing exclusive breastfeeding as the policy suggested, and weaning was as early as one month among some mothers. The finding supports the studies by Singh (2010) in Kumasi, Ghana, and Essien, Akpan, Ndebbio and John (2009) in a rural setting in Nigeria. This might be an indication that, mothers did not fully understand the rationale for most of the information they received on feeding practices. For example, mothers were not aware that lactating mothers are able to maintain adequate milk production largely independently of their nutritional status and body mass index. Breast milk production is unaffected by the mothers fluid intake. Several authors explained the importance of hydration and mother's well-being while breastfeeding, but an increase in water intake had no effect on building milk supply (Dearlove & Dearlove, 2005) and maintenance of lactation supply is dependent on response to demand and the more often the baby breastfeeds, the better will be the milk supply (Verralls, 2008).

Most ethnic groups in Ghana believe that soup, irrespective of the type, is a major booster of breast milk production. Light soup and palmnut soup are the most preferred by most ethnic groups. The midwives must therefore lay emphasis on the process of breast milk production as well so that mothers can intensify demand feeding. Furthermore, mothers were not aware that 90 percent of breast milk is water and 10 percent solid (Nagin, 2008) and that if more water is given to the baby it is likely that the baby's stomach may be full and may not have sufficient nutrients from breastfeeding.

Problems associated with period of weaning have been reported (Singh, 2010, Essien et al., 2009; Affram, 2013). The majority would start to give adult foods to their children at weaning (Affram, 2013). There are varieties of adult foods in Ghana. The common foods are mainly carbohydrate diets eaten with thickened spicy soups or stew, which may not be suitable for a child. Koko (maize porridge) has been identified as another weaning diet (Singh, 2010; Affram, 2013). However, it is a mere carbohydrate which may need additional protein to make it nutritious for the child otherwise the nutritional status of the child will be jeopardized.

With regard to the policy implementation Affram, (2013) found that the midwives have high knowledge on breastfeeding from the training they received from workshops on lactation management. They also have knowledge on breastfeeding from their basic midwifery education. However, they were not able to disseminate the right information to the mothers to fully implement the breast-feeding policy. The teaching methodology used by the midwives for the newly delivered mothers and the antenatal education regarding breastfeeding need to be re-organized. It was observed that important components of the policy were skipped, which deprived mothers of vital information for implementing the policy. Vital aspects in teaching such as demonstrations were ignored. There was no guide to follow and breastfeeding problems and their management were not discussed. Mothers, therefore, tend to go home with vague ideas about child feeding practices. At home, mothers and grandmothers may influence breastfeeding and before long, other foods are being introduced before the child is six months old and the consequences of that may be malnutrition, morbidity and death.

Social support is highly important for the success of breastfeeding. In Ghana all hospitals that are designated as baby friendly have mother-to-mother support groups trained for the community (IBFAN, 2006). According to Cattaneo, Yngue, Koletzko and Guzman (2004), in the Netherlands the mother-to-mother support groups have national coverage. Also in 13 European countries, peer counselors defined as lay (non-health professional) women were trained to provide individual support to mothers. The mother-to-mother support groups are funded or grant-aided and are otherwise supported by providers of regional or national health-care services. Women were made aware of the contact details and services were provided by these groups through newsletters, information sheets, telephone directories, and the internet. The function of mother-to-mother support is beneficial in the promotion of breastfeeding. The traditional support system that positively reinforced breastfeeding in the past is no longer in place and where modernization and bottle feeding has become the norm, mother-to-mother support becomes useful (Linkages, 2004).

The mother support groups in Mamprobi community were knowledgeable in what the breastfeeding policy entails. They were trained by the Ghana Infant Nutrition Action Network (GINAN) and prepared to support mothers in their communities. They were actively involved and working with zeal to assist many mothers to breastfeed at the initial stages of training. In addition, they were willing to continue with the same zeal they started with when they were enrolled. However, their major complaint was lack of assistance and support. An important finding was that unlike people from the European countries where the system is practiced and enhanced with national support, the mother-support system in Ghana is left without any help from the Ministry of Health or health personnel, and their duties were labeled as voluntary work. At the inception of their training, incentives were given to them from time to time and they were keen to assist mothers in the communities to fulfill the goals of the policy. With time these incentives were withdrawn and gradually, they in turn withdrew their services. Once there were no incentives they were no longer willing to assist and support the mothers in the communities (Affram, 2013). A lot of money was spent in training them and not making use of their knowledge as well as their services renders the training useless. The implication is that many mothers will continue to follow a varied of feeding practices leading to increase in child malnutrition, morbidity and mortality.

Factors Influencing Nutritional Status of Children

Several factors can influence the nutritional status of the child. Socio-demographic factors such as low economic status of mothers, mothers' education and environmental factors have been identified as determinant of nutritional status in the child (Rayhan and Khan, 2006; Wamani, Åstrøm, Peterson, Tumwine and Tylleskär, 2006). Appoh and Krekling (2005) found that mothers' nutritional knowledge irrespective of their educational level can have positive effect on children's nutrition.

A significant finding from the study of Affram (2013) was an observation of severe wasting (6.6 percent), babies thin for age (6.7 percent) and severely underweight (23.7 percent) among babies younger than six months. These results may reflect the feeding practices of the mothers. Malnutrition in children younger than six months can be attributed to absence of exclusive breastfeeding, inadequate teaching received regarding breastfeeding and the mothers feeding their children as they thought fit. Mothers can also be influenced by grandmothers and friends in child feeding practices. Low level of nutrition is associated with low immunity, and children are likely to have low resistance to common childhood diseases such as diarrhoea and respiratory tract infections which may lead to child mortality. Partial breastfeeding at an early age is detrimental to the growth of the child. The child's absorption and digestive system are not suitable for other foods (Dewey, 2001).

Affram (2013) found severe wasting among the age groups of 49-60 months, severe stunting between 13-24 months (10.1 percent) and 49-60 months (18.3 percent); and underweight 37-48 months (32.3 percent). This might be an indication of persistent deterioration of nutritional status of the children as they grow. Several factors may account for this. Children might be deprived of the necessary nutrients as a result of bad feeding practices from birth and consequently continue to falter as they grow. The age groups identified for high levels of wasting, stunting and underweight are the active stage when children really begin to run about and play. This is the time most of them start schooling. Apart from the need for energy, they need nutrients to build their body. Deprivation of good nutrition may account for the significant levels of malnutrition.

Breastfeeding and HIV-Positive Mothers

HIV can be transmitted during breastfeeding from an HIV-infected mother to her infant (WHO, 2008). Mother-to-child transmission (MTCT) is when an HIV-infected mother passes the virus to her baby. This can take place during pregnancy, labour and delivery or breastfeeding (WHO, 2008). In high-income countries, MTCT has been virtually eliminated as a result of effective voluntary counseling and testing (VCT) services, access to antiretroviral therapy, safe delivery practices and the availability and safe use of breast milk substitutes (Avert.Org, 2013). In these countries, some HIV-positive mothers may wish to breastfeed their infants. However, the advice from national health agencies is that they should avoid breastfeeding entirely due to the risk of HIV transmission which outweighs the risks associated with the use of infant formula.

There are ways to reduce the risk of transmission during breastfeeding. However, those approaches are not effective enough to recommend breastfeeding. Expert advice is that breastfeeding should be avoided if the mother is HIV-positive and other means of feeding her child are available. The United Nations recommends that mothers with HIV are advised not to breastfeed whenever the use of breast milk substitutes is acceptable, feasible, affordable, sustainable and safe (AFASS) (Ghana Health Service, 2006; WHO, 2010). However, where mothers live in areas where safe water is unavailable, then the risk of life-threatening conditions from replacement feeding may be higher than the risk from breastfeeding. Baby formula that is not given safely can make a baby very sick. For example, making formula with unclean water, or serving it in a bottle or cup that is not adequately clean can expose the baby to dangerous bacteria. Consequently, this can lead to infections, malnutrition and even death.

The WHO recommendations to HIV-positive mothers who choose to or are advised to breastfeed are based on whether a mother has access to antiretroviral drugs or not. If there is regular supply of antiretroviral drugs, she can exclusively breastfeed for the first six months of an infant's life and then introduces mix feeding until the infant is able to have a safe diet without breast milk if on antiretroviral drugs. Research indicates that, a combination of exclusive breastfeeding and the use of antiretroviral treatment can significantly reduce the risk of transmitting HIV to babies through breastfeeding (WHO, 2010). WHO further recommends that, HIV-positive mothers or their infants take antiretroviral drugs throughout the period of breastfeeding and until the infant is 12 months old. This suggests that they can benefit from breastfeeding with little risk of becoming infected. Mixed feeding (i.e. where breastfeeding is mixed with bottle feeding of water or formula, glucose water, gripe water, traditional medicine or other foods) is safe because the mother or infant is on antiretroviral drug.

In instances where a regular supply of antiretrovirals is not possible, mothers are advised to exclusively breastfeed for the first six months of an infant's life and wean to prevent mixed feeding. Mixed feeding is not advisable because it is believed that it carries higher risk than exclusive breastfeeding (Ghana Health Service, 2006). For example, formula feeding can irritate the lining of the baby's stomach or damage the lining of the stomach and intestines, thus making it easier for the HIV in breast milk to get in to cause infection (WHO, 2008). Following ingestion of HIV infected breast milk, the infant gut mucosal surfaces are the most likely site at which transmission can occur (WHO, 2008). However, the absence of ARVs should not necessarily be a contrain-dication for HIV-infected mothers to breastfeed where environmental and social circumstances are not safe or supportive of replacement feeding (WHO, 2010).

Challenges of Implementation of Breastfeeding Policy in Ghana

The implementation of the National Breastfeeding Policy in Ghana seemed to be have met many challenges. Among others is the influx of breast milk substitutes in the market under different brand names. This violates the recommendations of the International Code of Marketing of Breast-milk Substitutes adopted by Ghana (Ghana Health Service, 2000). Coupled with the misunderstanding of exclusive breastfeeding, mothers might gradually be shifting back to artificial feeding.

Mother support group activities may fade away if not supported and promoted. Breastfeeding mothers when left on their own will be influenced by grandmothers, friends, and non-health personnel and they may practice child feeding as they see fit, which can make it easier for malnutrition to persist. Working mothers are not getting enough support at their workplaces to fully implement the programme as maternity leave is generally still up to three months only and mothers may prefer to give breast milk substitutes to their children in their absence.

Future Prospects

The general state of feeding practices for children in Ghana needs to be improved. Liquids such as water and juice and even solid foods are given to children earlier than the recommended age of six months. This practice has a deleterious effect on the nutritional status of the child. The trends of exclusive breastfeeding policy implementation seemed to be on the decline. There is general awareness among the public but many mothers might not actually be practicing exclusive breastfeeding. If intervention programmes are not put in place very soon, exclusive breastfeeding will be a thing of the past and the goal for the policy may not be achieved. There is the need for major a survey by the Ministry of Health and Ghana Health Service to identify problems affecting the breastfeeding policy at each implementation stage and corrective measures put in place, otherwise malnutrition and infant mortality may still remain high and exclusive breastfeeding remain a distant objective in Ghana.

Recommendations

- The work of mother support groups must be recognised and duly rewarded so that they continue to support mothers in the community and help to improve the lives of children.
- The government must provide logistics and teaching aids on breastfeeding in all health institutions.
- The laws on the use of breastfeeding substitutes must be enforced and the enthusiasm with which initial enforcement of the law was greeted must prevail at all times.

- All public health nurses must have training in midwifery before being accepted into community health institutions so that they can appreciate the importance of pregnancy, childbirth and care of children because this group of nurses continues to supervise mothers after six weeks of delivery throughout the weaning periods of the child and subsequent years.

Conclusion

The National Breastfeeding Policy implementation was instituted to decrease childhood malnutrition, morbidity and mortality. Numerous problems concerning the implementation of the policy at various levels pose challenges for its success. The nursing mothers may not grasp the meaning of exclusive breastfeeding if they are not receiving the right information to implement proper child feeding. They will be left to the influence and decisions of relatives as to what to feed their children and when. Mothers' feeding practices may worsen further if the support groups promoting exclusive breastfeeding are no longer active. The market is also flooded with attractive breast milk substitutes and feeding bottles. This is a hindrance to full implementation of the policy. Unless measures are put in place to overcome the challenges facing the implementation of the National Breastfeeding Policy, the aims of the policy cannot be achieved and child morbidity and mortality might remain high.

References

Affram, C.K. (2013). *Implementation of the National Breastfeeding Policy in Ghana*. Unpublished manuscript.

Avert.Org. (2013). *Preventing mother-to-child transmission of HIV*. Available at: http://www.avert.org /motherchild.htm. [Accessed on 29 May 2013].

Appoh, L.Y., & Krekling, S. (2005). Maternal nutritional knowledge and child nutritional status in the Volta Region of Ghana. *Blackwell Publishing Ltd Maternal and Child Nutrition*, 1, 100-110. Available at: www. ghana. gov.gh/index.php?option breastfeeding-in-Ghana. [Accessed on: 1 February 2010].

Cattaneo, A., Yngue, B., Koletzko, L., & Guzman, R. (2004). Protection, Promotion and Support of Breast-Feeding in Europe: Current Situation. *Public Health Nutrition*, 8(1), 39-46.

Dearlove, J.C. & Dearlove, B.M. (2005). Prolactin, fluid balance and lactation. *BJOG: An International Journal of Obstetrics & Gynaecology*, 88(6):652-654. DOI: 10.1111/j.1471-05228.1981.tb01225.x (accessed on 27/05/2013).

Dewey, K. (2001). Guiding principles for complementary feeding of the breastfed. Available at: www. ghana.gov.gh/index.php?option breast-feeding-in-Ghana. [Accessed on: 1 February 2010].

Essien, N.C., Akpan, P.E., Ndebbio, T.J., & John, M.E. (2009). Mothers' knowledge, attitudes, beliefs and practices concerning exclusive breastfeeding in Calabar, Nigeria, *Africa Journal on Nursing and Midwifery*, 11 (1), 65-75.

Frost, M.B., Forste, R. & Hass, D.W. (2004). Maternal education and child nutritional status in Bolivia. *Social Science & Medicine*, 60 (2005), 395-407.

Infant Baby Food Action Network (2006). Ghana Country Report. 7th Infant Baby Food Action Network (IBFAN) Africa Regional conference.

Ghana Health Service. (2000). *Breastfeeding Promotion Regulation, 2000*. (LI 1667).

Ghana Health Service. (2004). Reproductive and Child Health Unit, *Annual report*

Ghana Health Service. (2006). *Guidelines on nutritional care and support for people living with HIV and AIDS*. Accra: Konsept Design.

Ghana Statistical Service. (2008). *Ghana Demographic and Health Survey*: Fact Sheet. Accra: GSS.

Grigsby, D.G. (2006). *Malnutrition eMedicine*. Available at: www.emedicine.com/ped/topic/1360.htm. [Accessed: 1 November 2008].

Kramer, M.S., & Kakuma, R. (2002). Optimal duration of exclusive breast-feeding. *Cochrane Database of Systematic Reviews*, Issue 1. Art. No.: CD003517.D01: 10.1002/14651858.CD003517.

Linkages. (2004). *Mother-to-mother support for breastfeeding frequently asked questions*. Available at: www.tensteps.org/breastfeeding-fag- mother-mother-support [Accessed: 1 November 2009].

Maurice, K., Saloojee, H. and Westwood, T. (2008). *Child health for all*. 4th ed. Cape Town: Oxford University Press.

Ministry of Health Ghana. (2006). *Multiple Indicator Cluster Survey*. Accra

Nagin, M.K. (2008). Breast milk content and composition of breast milk. Available at: http://breastfeedingabout.com/od/breastfeedingbasics/p/bmcontent. ht[Accessed on 1 March 2012].

Rayham, Md. I. & Khan, M.S. (2006). Factors causing malnutrition among under-five children in Angladesh, Pakistan. *Journal of Nutrition*, 5(6), 556-562.

Senbanjo, I.O., Adeodu, O.O., & Adejuyigbe, E.A. (2007). Low prevalence of malnutrition in a rural Nigerian community. *Tropical Doctor*, 37: 214-216.

Singh, B. (2010). Knowledge, attitude and practice of breast feeding – A case study. *European Journal of Scientific Research*, 40(3), 404-422.

Verrals, S. (2008). *Anatomy and Physiology Applied to Obstetrics*. Toronto: Churchill Livingstone.

Wamani, H. et al. (2006). Predictors of poor anthropometric status among children under 2 years of age in rural Uganda. *Public Health Nutrition*, 9(3), 320-326.

Weimer, J.P. (1999). *Breastfeeding: health and economic issues*. Available at: www.ers.usda.gov/publications/foodreview/may1999/frmay99h.pdf. [Accessed: 30 November 2009].

WHO. (2001a). *Measuring child mortality*. Available at: www.who.int/child_adolescent health/data/child/eb/index.html [Accessed: 12 October 2009].

WHO. (2001b). *The optimal duration of exclusive breastfeeding: Report of an expert consultation*. Geneva: World Health Organisation.

WHO. (2008). *HIV transmission through breastfeeding: a review of available evidence – An update from 2001 to 2007*. Paris: WHO Press.

WHO. (2010). *Guidelines on HIV and infant feeding 2010: Principles and recommendations for infants feeding in the context of HIV and a summary of evidence*. Geneva: WHO Press.

WHO. (2013). *Promoting proper feeding for infants and young children*. Geneva. Available at: www.who.int/nutrition/topics/infantfeeding/en/. [Accessed: 26 May 2013].

Chapter Eight
Female Infertility and its Management in Ghana: Emerging Concerns and Strategies

Florence Naab and Ernestina S. Donkor

Introduction

In 2001, the World Health Organization (WHO) pronounced infertility a worldwide public health issue because of the global challenges associated with the availability and accessibility of infertility treatment and assisted reproduction, which in many ways, may affect the health outcomes of infertile women (WHO, 2001). What is known about infertility differs according to whether infertility is identified by self-report, based on a life calendar of reproductive events, or a physician consultation and diagnosis (Fisher, 2009). For instance, in high-income countries, infertility is often associated with the late start of child bearing (WHO, 2009). As a result, the definition of infertility has a significant impact on clinical outcomes and thus, infertility can be regarded as a heterogeneous group of health problems (Fisher, 2009).

Infertility is generally defined as the inability to conceive after at least one year of regular and unprotected sexual intercourse (Oko-nofua, Harris, Odebiyi, Kane, & Snow, 1997). Medically, infertility is classified as primary or secondary. It is primary when the couple has had no previous pregnancy and secondary if they have had a previous pregnancy irrespective of the outcome of the pregnancy (Kwawukume & Emuveyan, 2005). Thus, estimation of the prevalence rate of infertility depends on how infertility is defined (Fisher, 2009).

Based on the medical definition of infertility, international estimates are that, 72.4 million women in the world are infertile (Boivin, Bunting, Collins, & Nygren, 2007). Out of this population, it is reported that most women with infertility live in the developing world (WHO, 2009). Furthermore, with as many as 80 million people suffering involuntary childlessness worldwide, infertility has become a global reproductive health problem (Nachtigall, 2006). In sub-Saharan Africa, the prevalence rates for infertility vary from 20 percent to 48 percent (Kwawukume & Emuveyan, 2005), with about 30 percent of couples suffering primary or secondary infertility (WHO, 2009). The prevalence rates in sub-Saharan Africa are relatively high within a common age range. For instance, of women aged 20 to 44 years, the prevalence rates of secondary infertility are: 20 percent in Cameroon, 25 percent in Lesotho, 21 percent each in Mozambique and Mauritania (Boivin et al., 2007). Although the prevalence of infertility in Ghana is 16 percent for women aged 20 to 44 years (Larsen, 2000), this report is more than a decade old and no new data are currently available. Comparatively, while the prevalence of infertility among sub-Saharan African couples with primary or secondary infertility is about 30 percent, it is 28 percent in South-Central Asia and 24 percent in South-East Asia (WHO, 2009). These prevalence rates seem to suggest that the management of infertility in the whole of sub-Saharan Africa needs to be evaluated.

Infertility as a Women's Health Problem in Ghana

In most African societies, where child bearing is highly valued (Barden-O'Fallon, 2005; de Kok and Widdicombe, 2008; Runganga, Sundby, & Aggleton, 2001), infertility is associated with psychosocial health problems such as stress, anxiety and depression (Donkor & Sandall, 2007; Dyer, Abrahams, Hoffman, & Van der Spuy, 2002a; Dyer, Abrahams, Mokoena, Lombard, & van der Spuy, 2005; Naab, 2012; Upkong & Orji, 2006). Given the high prevalence rates of infertility in sub-Saharan Africa, its psychosocial health outcomes have been reported in the areas of psychological distress, and social health problems. Research in the area of women's infertility-related psychosocial health problems is discussed in detail below.

Psychological Distress Outcomes of Infertility

Psychological distress has been reported among infertile African women. In South Africa, Dyer and colleagues found that infertile women as compared to fertile women reported higher levels of psychological distress such as anxiety and depression as a result of physical, emotional, and verbal abuse by their husbands (Dyer et al., 2005). Similarly, a study in Nigeria found that 37.5 percent and 42.9 percent of infertile women (N=112) reported high levels of anxiety and depression respectively (Upkong & Orji, 2006). These authors also reported that women with primary infertility had significantly higher anxiety and depression scores than women with secondary infertility. Furthermore, when Fatoye, Owolabi, Eegunranti, and Fatoye (2008) compared anxiety and depressive symptoms between infertile Nigerian women (N=82) and their husbands (N=82), more women (40.2 percent) had higher levels of anxiety than their husbands (20.7 percent), and more women (42.7 percent) were depressed than their husbands (15.9 percent). Even though the study did not examine any factors that might explain the gender differences in anxiety and depression among couples, the authors recommended the need for attitudinal change to improve the emotional health of infertile couples.

In Ghana, a number of studies have reported psychological distress among infertile women. In 2007, Donkor & Sandall reported infertility-related stress and stigma among women seeking infertility treatment in southern Ghana (Donkor, & Sandall, 2007). Specifically, the authors reported that 23 percent of the women experienced moderate stigma and 41 percent experienced severe infertility-related perceived stigma while women who reported severe levels of perceived stigma had the highest mean score for infertility-related stress. Furthermore, two recent studies in Ghana reported the mental health effects of infertility among Ghanaian women (Fledderjohann, 2012; Naab, 2012). Infertile Ghanaian women have reported many psychosocial consequences such as social stigma, marital instability, and mental health problems including worrying, crying for long periods, and insomnia (Fledderjohann, 2012). Similarly, 53 percent of women (N = 203) seeking treatment for fertility problems in Ghana were clinically depressed (Naab, 2012). Similar experiences have been reported among South African infertile women with involuntary childlessness, including burning pain, anger, deep sadness, bitterness, guilt, loneliness, and desperation as psychological suffering (Dyer et al., 2002a). Consequently, infertility among Ghanaian women may be described as a crisis that needs intervention for the mental health safety of these women.

Social Health Outcomes of Infertility

Negative consequences of infertility, such as divorce, abandonment, social isolation, stigmatization, abuse, and social pressure have been reported in Nigeria. For instance, full adult status among women is only attainable through marriage and child birth, and a childless married woman is described as a man because of her inability to bear children (Hollos, Larsen, Obono, & Whitehouse, 2009). The authors also reported some social consequences such as infertility being a good reason for a man to marry a second wife; in old age, an infertile woman is not cared for, and in death an infertile woman cannot be buried on town land, since it is believed that this could harm the land's fertility (Hollos et al., 2009). In Zimbabwe, Runganga and colleagues (2001) reported some beliefs which may also contribute to the social suffering of infertile African women. Beliefs such as life without children is "just life without any purpose", "childbearing offers women a sense of womanhood", and that children are a "source of emotional security" for women have been reported (Runganga et al., 2001, p. 327). Furthermore, the women reported being isolated from other women and not allowed to contribute to discussions about children or advise on ways to solve problems related to children. A commonly held belief reported by the women was that "if a marriage is childless, it lacks the dignity of a real family" (Runganga et al., 2001, p. 327) which may imply that a marriage is incomplete without children. The authors concluded that because women bear the burden for childlessness in a couple, women experience considerable social distress. These social distress consequences appear to be detrimental to the mental health of these women.

In Ghana, the impact of social distress on the mental health of infertile women is not different. Infertile women are reported to be socially isolated in their communities (Fledderjohann, 2012). Yet, there is no evidence of any intervention for the psychosocial health needs of infertile women in Ghana.

Management of infertility in Ghana

Although the infertility literature in Africa indicates that the experience of infertility affects the mental health of women, infertility is rarely recognized as a serious health problem that requires a combination of medical and psychological treatment. As a result, the treatment of infertility is mainly medical with a focus on ovulatory stimulation and assisted reproductive treatment [ART] in some countries (Nachtigall, 2006; Sharma, Mittal, & Aggarwal, 2009; Ombelet, Cooke, Dyer, Serour, & Devroey, 2008; Van Balen & Gerrits, 2001). However, ART is cost prohibitive for many infertile women in Africa (Nachtigall, 2006). Thus, the management of infertility generally involves ovulatory stimulation with drugs, surgical techniques, and ART.

Ovulatory stimulation or induction is indicated when laboratory investigations show evidence of ovulatory dysfunction. The most common drug used for ovulatory induction is clomiphene citrate which has an ovulation achievement rate of about 70 percent and with timed intercourse, achieves pregnancy in about 25 percent per cycle (Sharma et al., 2009). Gonadotrophins (hormones secreted by the anterior pituitary gland) may also be used to induce ovulation although Sharma and colleagues (2009) cautioned that gonado-trophins may predispose the woman to ovarian hyper-stimulation syndrome (OHSS).

Surgical techniques used to resolve tubal blockage are reported to have a success rate of about 50 percent (Sharma et al., 2009). Even though the success rate of surgical techniques for tubal blockage may be encouraging, this option is not available in most developing countries because of the cost involved in tubal surgery. It is therefore sad to note that, despite the fact that the prevalence rates of infertility are high in sub-Saharan Africa, tubal surgery with its high success rate may not be an option for sub-Saharan African infertile women.

The use of ART is widespread in Africa (Nachtigall, 2006; Sharma et al., 2009; Ombelet et al., 2008; Van Balen & Gerrits, 2001) but may not be affordable for the average African woman because of the cost involved. Unfortunately, it is estimated that, of all couples who seek infertility treatment, up to about 10 percent will require some form of

ART (Sharma et al., 2009). Hence, there is no doubt that the treatment of infertility may be a source of stress to women, especially those of low socio-economic status. As a result, the treatment of infertility in Africa needs to be evaluated because of the cost and the involvement of other psychosocial problems such as stress and depression among women.

In Ghana, the management of women with infertility is not different. Infertile women are subjected to only medical treatment while the psychosocial health problems such as depression go untreated. Therefore, there is the need to add some form of psycho-educational counseling to the medical treatment. This addition will provide holistic healthcare of infertile women in Ghana.

Emerging Concerns of Infertility

The emerging concerns involving the management of infertility are research-related concerns, mental health problems resulting from being infertile, lack of psycho-educational counseling for victims of infertility, and religious/spirituality-related influence.

Research-Related Concerns

Many of the research-related concerns are methodological. For instance, the most common research design for studies on the social and psychological consequences of infertility is cross-sectional, which makes it difficult to sort out the actual effects of infertility on health outcomes. The use of longitudinal designs to study the impact of infertility on women's health in Africa is yet to be done. Another methodological concern lies in the types of samples recruited for infertility studies. The sample is mostly clinic-based. Clinic-based studies tend to recruit only treatment seekers, thereby making it difficult to generalize the findings to infertile women who are not seeking treatment. Because many studies in Africa use clinic-based samples predominantly, there is a proliferation of reports about poor psychosocial health outcomes of infertile women. Meanwhile, the stress of undergoing infertility treatment alone may influence how much stress, anxiety, or depression is experienced by these women. Thus, the clinic-based samples may be the explanation for the unusually higher mean scores on anxiety, stress and depression among infertile African women because in the Western world, studies have demonstrated positive correlations between infertility treatment and psychosocial distress (Abbey, Halman, & Andrews, 1992; Schneider & Forthofer, 2005). Therefore, clinic-based samples have the potential to score high in psychosocial distress and may provide little information about the total population of infertile women. To counteract this flaw, however, studies using clinic-based samples need to examine other possible explanations for psychosocial distress rather than using infertility diagnosis to predict psychosocial distress.

The measures used to quantify infertility-related psychosocial distress constitute another type of methodological issue of concern. Studies in Africa have used measures such as the hospital anxiety and depression scale (HADS), Beck's depression inventory, and fertility problem inventory to estimate infertility-related psychosocial distress. Many of these measures may lack cultural appropriateness in Africa. Therefore, these measures may require some modification to fit the culture of the people being studied. The HADS is a measure that has been used extensively to measure infertility-related anxiety and depression in Africa. However, the failure to modify the measure may lead to participant misunderstanding. For instance, "I get sudden feelings of panic", is one of the items in the HADS. The understanding of this item in an African sample may vary from one African language to another. For example, among the Dagaaba of northern Ghana, "sudden feelings of panic" may be understood as fear because there is no known word for "panic" (anecdotal report).

In summary, the inconsistencies in the findings of infertility research in Africa may largely be due to methodological problems such as the reliance on small, non-representative samples, clinic-based samples of treatment seekers, use of cross-sectional designs, and the use of general rather than specific measures to quantify infertility-related psycho-social distress. Fortunately, these problems have been recognized in the literature and researchers in the US and other developed countries have begun addressing them (Greil, Slauson-Blevins, & McQuillan, 2010). However, there is no evidence of these problems being addressed in Africa. There is a need for a critical review of the infertility literature in Africa to examine if these issues are being addressed. Addressing these issues may lead to evidence-based research findings which will improve the management of infertility for African women.

Mental Health Problems Resulting from Infertility

A review of the infertility literature in Africa suggests that infertile women in Africa have some mental health problems (Dyer, Abrahams, Hoffman, & van der Spuy, 2002b; Fatoye, Owolabi, Eegunranti, & Fatoye, 2008; Upkong & Orji, 2006). For instance, cases of women's infertility-related poor mental health have been reported in Nigeria (Upkong & Orji, 2006), in South Africa, (Dyer et al., 2002b), and in Ghana (Donkor & Sandall, 2007; Fledderjohann, 2012; Naab, 2012). However, the management of infertility in Africa is primarily medical and does not include the management of mental health problems. This situation begs the question as to whether the mental health problems that are empirically reported are neglected and ignored. It is evident that infertile women in Africa have mental health problems that need some psycho-educational intervention.

Lack of Psycho-Educational Counseling/ Intervention

Psycho-educational intervention is a combination of educational or teaching activities and psychological activities (Hawley, 1995). The goal of psycho-educational intervention is to alter outcomes by facilitating voluntary adaptations of behaviour and increasing knowledge (Hawley, 1995). In the USA, there is a social support group known as Resolve which offers several avenues of
support including familiarity with the latest treatments, strategies for coping with specific sources of crisis, and the formation of various support groups. According to Parry (2005), women in the Resolve groups read and learn about their infertility, which enables the women to play active roles in the decision-making process affecting their infertility. Thus, the knowledge acquired by these women about their infertility empowers them to make informed decisions and choices.

In Africa, data on psycho-educational counseling for infertile women are non-existent. This means that even though most infertile women in Africa have psychosocial health problems, psycho-educational counseling has never been considered as a complement for the management of infertility. A recent study in Ghana showed that Ghanaian women with infertility reported a lack of knowledge about their infertility (Naab, 2012), which suggests that psycho-educational counseling or intervention would be beneficial to this group of women. However, in Ghana, the psycho-educational needs of infertile women are yet to be given the needed attention. Therefore, in addition to medical treatment, psycho-educational counseling will be a step in the right direction to managing the psychosocial health problems of infertile women in Ghana.

Religious/Spirituality-Related Influence

In Ghana, apart from biomedical causes of infertility, traditional or religious causes of infertility such as witchcraft have been cited (Donkor & Sandall, 2012). Consequently, in the treatment of infertility, many women resort to traditional healing and spiritual mediation (including churches) in addition to orthodox medicine (Donkor & Sandall, 2012; Dyer et al., 2002b). Some women are deeply convinced of supernatural causes, and so they patronize the services of traditional and religious healers for spiritual help. In Ghana today, it is common to see many women testifying in churches to the fact that they have been able to conceive through prayers. However, it is not clear if these spiritual/religious remedies are able to mitigate women's psychosocial health problems such as depression.

The Role of the Nurse in the Care of Women with Infertility in Ghana

The role of the nurse in the management of infertility among women is twofold. First, nurses can provide health education for women with fertility problems. Secondly, nurses also need to explore infertility with empirical research. It is reported that infertile Ghanaian women lack knowledge about their infertility (Naab, 2012) and this lack of knowledge may contribute to the high levels of stress and depression among Ghanaian infertile women (Donkor & Sandall, 2007; Naab, 2012). As a result, it will be appropriate for nurses to provide these women with the necessary medical information related to their infertility to help reduce the levels of stress and depression among them. Areas such as the causes of infertility, available treatment for infertility, and the need to see a psychologist for mental health counseling should be emphasized during health education for these women. Furthermore, Ghanaian women have reported many negative beliefs about infertility, some of which are not medically correct (Naab, 2012). It is only through health education that nurses may be able to demystify some of these beliefs, by replacing the negative beliefs with the appropriate medical information.

Research in the area of psychosocial health problems of women with infertility has not been well explored. For instance, women's beliefs about infertility account for their levels of anxiety, stress, stigma, social isolation, and depression (Naab, 2012). Yet, little is known about the predictors of these psychosocial health problems. Therefore, until recently, scientific evidence which is needed to provide mental health care for women with infertility was almost non-existent. There is a need for nurse researchers in Ghana and Africa as a whole, to explore this area and provide evidence through intervention research for appropriate care of women with infertility in Ghana.

Conclusion

Infertility is a global reproductive health problem. In Africa where childbearing is highly valued among women, infertility may be described and experienced as a crisis. Research has shown that infertile women in Ghana report psychological, social, and mental health problems. These reports suggest the need for psychosocial management of these problems. However, the management of infertility in Ghana is primarily medical. As a result, the psychosocial or mental health needs of these women have never been addressed. Thus, the issue of infertility brings to light many emerging concerns including research-related concerns, mental health problems lack of psycho-educational counseling and religious/spirituality-related influence. Further research addressing the existing gaps in the literature is needed to examine other factors rather than the mere diagnosis that contributes to the psychosocial distress among infertile women. The value of children in Ghana makes women's experience of infertility more mental health-related and signifies the need for psycho-educational counseling for these women.

References

Abbey, A., Halman, L. J., & Andrews, F. M. (1992). Psychosocial, treatment, and demographic predictors of the stress associated with infertility. *Fertility & Sterility.* 57(1), 122-128.

Barden-O'Fallon, J. (2005). Unmet fertility expectations and the perception of fertility problems in a Malawian village. *African Journal of Reproductive Health*, 14–25.

Boivin, J., Bunting, L., Collins, J. A., & Nygren, K. G. (2007). International estimates of infertility prevalence and treatment-seeking: potential need and demand for infertility medical care. *Human Reproduction*, 22(6), 1506-1512.

de Kok, B. C., & Widdicombe, S. (2008). 'I really tried': Management of normative issues in accounts of infertility. *Social Science & Medicine*, 67(7), 1083–1093.

Donkor, E. S., & Sandall, J. (2007).The impact of perceived stigma and mediating social factors on infertility-related stress among women seeking infertility treatment in Southern Ghana. *Social Science & Medicine*, 65(8), 1683–1694.

Donkor, E. S., and Sandall, J. (2012). *Perceived stigma, stress and coping strategies among infertile women.* USA: Lap Lambert Academic Publishing.

Dyer, S. J., Abrahams, N., Hoffman, M., & van der Spuy, Z. M. (2002a). 'Men leave me as I cannot have children': women's experiences with involuntary childlessness. *Human Reproduction*, 17(6), 1663-1668.

Dyer, S., Abrahams, N., Hoffman, M., & Van der Spuy, Z. (2002b). Infertility in South Africa: women's reproductive health knowledge and treatment-seeking behaviour for involuntary childlessness. *Human Reproduction*, 17(6), 1657-1662.

Dyer, S. J., Abrahams, N., Mokoena, N., Lombard, C. J., & van der Spuy, Z. M. (2005). Psychological distress among women suffering from couple infertility in South Africa: a quantitative assessment. *Human Reproduction*, 20(7), 1938-1943.

Fatoye, F., Owolabi, A., Eegunranti, B., & Fatoye, G. (2008). Unfulfilled desire for pregnancy: Gender and family differences in emotional burden among a Nigerian sample. *Journal of Obstetrics & Gynecology*, 28(4), 408–409.

Fisher, J. (2009). *Infertility and assisted reproduction. Mental health aspects of women's reproductive health. A global review of the literature.* Geneva: World Health Organization, pp. 128-146.

Fledderjohann, J. J. (2012). 'Zero is not good for me': implications of infertility in Ghana. *Human Reproduction.* Available at: http://humrep. oxfordjournals.org/content/early/2012/02/21/humrep.des035.short

Greil, A. L., Slauson-Blevins, K., & McQuillan, J. (2010). The experience of infertility: a review of recent literature. *Sociology of Health & Illness*, 32(1), 140–162.

Hawley, D. J. (1995). Psycho-educational interventions in the treatment of arthritis. *Baillière's clinical rheumatology*, 9(4), 803–823.

Hollos, M., Larsen, U., Obono, O., & Whitehouse, B. (2009). The problem of infertility in high fertility populations: meanings, consequences and coping mechanisms in two Nigerian communities. *Social Science & Medicine*, 68(11), 2061–2068.

Kwawukume, E., & Emuveyan, E. (2005). *Comprehensive Gynecology in the Tropics.* Accra: Graphic Packging Ltd.

Larsen, U. (2000). Primary and secondary infertility in sub-Saharan Africa. *International Journal of Epidemiology*, 29(2), 285.

Naab, F. (2012). Women's representations of infertility in Ghana. Dissertation research. The University of Wisconsin-Madison *ProQuest,* UMI Number: 3489069.

Nachtigall, R. D. (2006). International disparities in access to infertility services. *Fertility and Sterility*, 85(4), 871–875.

Okonofua, F., Harris, D., Odebiyi, A., Kane, T., & Snow, R. C. (1997). The social meaning of infertility in Southwest Nigeria. *Health Transition Review*, 7, 205–220.

Ombelet, W., Cooke, I., Dyer, S., Serour, G., & Devroey, P. (2008). Infertility and the provision of infertility medical services in developing countries. *Human Reproduction Update*, 14(6), 605–621.

Parry, D. C. (2005). Women's experiences with infertility: Exploring the outcome of empowerment. *Women's Studies*, 34(2), 191–211.

Runganga, A. O., Sundby, J., & Aggleton, P. (2001). Culture, identity and reproductive failure in Zimbabwe. *Sexualities*, 4(3), 315-332.

Schneider, M. G., & Forthofer, M. S. (2005). Associations of psychosocial factors with the stress of infertility treatment. *Health and Social Work*, 30(3), 183–191.

Sharma, S., Mittal, S., & Aggarwal, P. (2009). Management of infertility in low-resource countries. *BJOG: An International Journal of Obstetrics & Gynaecology*, 116, 77–83.

Upkong, D., & Orji, E. (2006). Mental health of infertile women in Nigeria. *Turk Psikiyatri Dergisi*, 17(4), 259-265.

Van Balen, F., & Gerrits, T. (2001). Quality of infertility care in poor-resource areas and the introduction of new reproductive technologies. *Human Reproduction*, 16(2), 215.

World Health Organization. (2001). *Global prevalence and incidence of selected curable sexually transmitted infections: overview and estimates*. Geneva: World Health Organization.

World Health Organization. (2009). *Women and health: Today's evidence, tomorrow's agenda*. Geneva: World Health Organization.

Chapter Nine
Curbing Unsafe Abortions in Ghana: Policy Implications and Stakeholders' Concerns

Patience Aniteye

Introduction

Unsafe abortion (and the associated morbidity and mortality in women) is preventable yet it constitutes a great challenge for women's reproductive health in sub-Saharan Africa (Okonofua, 2004). It is a significant cause of the persistently high maternal mortality ratios in the region (Hessini, Brookman–Amissah, & Crane, 2006). Most African countries have restrictive abortion laws which they inherited from pre-independence colonial laws of France, England, Belgium and Portugal. Although most of these countries have amended their laws, their former colonies still hold on to these laws which can even restrict the provision of abortion services to save women's lives (Ngwena, 2004). Even where abortion laws have been liberalized, the formulation of policies to translate such laws into services has been a protracted process. Some socio-cultural and service-related factors impinge on the availability of safe abortion services (Okonofua, 2004). There are also strong debates for and against the provision of abortion services among key stakeholders which influence availability of services. This chapter discusses the measures aimed at preventing unsafe abortion, and the legal and policy implications. The introduction of comprehensive abortion care (CAC) in public health facilities in Ghana and the concerns raised by this measure are also presented.

The Global Burden of Unsafe Abortion

Each year, all around the world, about 210 million women become pregnant. As many as 80 million pregnancies are unintended, resulting mainly from contraceptive non-use, inconsistent or incorrect use of contraceptives or both, contraceptive failure or poor access to contraceptives. Some of these pregnancies are carried to term, while others end in spontaneous or induced abortion. Induced abortions have been carried out for a long time all over the world. Abortion is a controversial issue in reproductive health and it is characterized by stigma and criminalization as well as moral and religious condemnation (Lithur, 2004; Mundigo & Indriso, 1999). Due to the controversial and sensitive nature of abortion, its incidence as well as abortion-related morbidity and mortality are difficult to establish. It is estimated that 46 million pregnancies are deliberately terminated each year-27 million legally and 19 million outside the legal system (WHO, 2004). Current estimates by the WHO (2012) put the global number of unsafe abortions each year at 22 million. According to estimates by Sedgh, Singh, Henshaw and Bankole (2007), the global figure for induced abortion decreased from 46 million in 1995 to 42 million in 2003. They further observed that between 1995 and 2003, the induced abortion rate decreased from 35 to 29 per 1,000 women aged 15-44. The decrease in abortion rates was more marked in high-income than in low- and middle-income (LMIC) countries. Even though the overall incidence and rate of induced abortion declined worldwide between 1995 and 2003, the proportion of unsafe abortions increased from 44 percent to 48 percent with the vast majority occurring in low- and middle-income countries. Recent estimates indicated that the global abortion rate remained stable between 2003 and 2008. The abortion rates were 29 and 28 abortions per 1,000 women aged 15-44 respectively and about 49 percent of abortions were unsafe in 2008 (Sedgh et al., 2012).

Estimates of Unsafe Abortion

Unsafe abortion has been defined as a procedure for terminating an unwanted pregnancy either by persons lacking the necessary skills or in an environment lacking the minimal medical standards or both (WHO, 2012; Ahman & Shah, 2004). Unsafe abortions are usually performed by unskilled providers who use dangerous techniques in facilities lacking proper sanitation. They constitute a major neglected reproductive health problem in low- and middle-income countries (WHO, 1998, 2004). The procedure exacts a heavy toll on women's lives all over the world. Data on unsafe abortions are particularly difficult to obtain since most of them happen outside legally provided services and are therefore not officially recorded (Ahiadeke, 2001). Of the 20-22 million unsafe abortions that occur each year in the world about 47,000 result in death and 5 million women are maimed as a result of complications (WHO, 2011, 2012). Furthermore, WHO (2012) maintains that about 98 percent of the unsafe abortions that occur in the world, occur in low- and middle-income countries (LMIC) under illegal conditions. It estimate that the death rate from unsafe abortion in Africa is 100/100,000 live births and considers it to be the highest in the world. In the US, the death rate from abortion is 0.6/100,000 (Raymond & Grimes, 2012). WHO (2012) noted that death from unsafe abortion is the easiest to prevent of all the causes of maternal mortality and concluded that reducing unwanted pregnancies in Africa would reduce the number of deaths from unsafe abortion.

Unsafe abortion is a very common experience in Africa (Braam and Hessini 2004; Hord & Wolf, 2004). Women in sub-Saharan Africa face the highest risk of death and injury from abortion complications worldwide and 43 percent of the 68,000 women who die from these complications each year are from Africa (Hessini, Brookman–Amissah, & Crane, 2006). Recent studies in Kenya, Uganda and Nigeria of women in public health facilities with complications from unsafe abortion show the magnitude of the burden of unsafe abortion which Hessini et al. (2006) describe as a public health crisis, a social injustice and a violation of women's human rights and dignity.

Unsafe Abortion in Ghana

The Ghana Maternal Health Survey (GMHS, 2007) shows that at least 7 percent of all pregnancies in Ghana end in abortion, and 15 percent of women aged 15–49 admitted to having had an abortion. Abortion rates were highest among 20–24-year-olds, educated and wealthier women, and those living in urban areas. The survey further indicated that just over half of Ghanaian women who admitted having had an abortion sought help from a doctor, while others turned to pharmacists or traditional midwives to induce abortion. Almost one in five women induced the abortion themselves or had the help of a friend. Although abortion is legal in Ghana under certain conditions, unsafe abortion is still thought to make a significant contribution to the burden of maternal morbidity and mortality, especially among adolescents (Aboagye, Gebreselassie, Quansah Asare, Mitchell & Addy, 2007; Mayhew, 2004). Ghana's maternal mortality stands at 580 per 100,000 live births (GMHS, 2007). Complications from unsafe abortion are thought to constitute 22 to 30 percent of all maternal deaths, thus making unsafe abortion the highest contributor to maternal mortality in Ghana (Aboagye & Akosa, 2000; Ghana Health Service, 2004-2008). Other sources indicate that unsafe abortion contributes 12 percent to 15 percent of maternal mortality in Ghana (Baird, Billings, & Demuyakor, 2000; Geelhoed, Visser, Asare, Schagen van Leeuwen, & van Roosmalen, 2003; Ministry of Health and Ghana Statistical Service, 2003). These discrepancies make data on abortion unreliable.

According to Ahiadeke (2001), data on abortion in Ghana are generally scarce, fragmented and unreliable. He observes that most studies on induced abortion in Ghana are hospital-based; that all but one of the 22 studies on abortion carried out between 1972 and 1994 were hospital-based and as many as 19 took place in Korle Bu Teaching Hospital, Ghana's largest teaching hospital. In his view, since induced abortion is perceived as illegal in the Ghanaian context, women admitted to hospital with complications of induced abortion are likely to be documented as women hospitalized with complications from spontaneous abortion. He identified factors such as poor record-keeping, inaccurate classification of type of abortions done by doctors and the lack of policies that demand accurate classification of abortion as accounting for unreliable data on induced abortion and also making hospital data inadequate for estimating Ghana's nation-wide incidence of induced abortion. In his study on the incidence of induced abortion in southern Ghana (one of the few community-based studies in Ghana), there were 27 abortions for every 100 live births. The vast majority of the women who had an abortion (60%) were younger than

30; about one-third of women obtained an abortion from within the health system while the remaining 68% reported having obtained an abortion from pharmacists (38%), by self medication (11%), from an untrained provider (16%) or by other means (3%).

In terms of morbidity, unsafe abortion exacts a heavy toll. It leads to complications such as infection, profuse bleeding, perforated womb, and damage to internal organs (Grimes et al. 2006, WHO 2004). In Ghana, studies have documented similar complications (Adanu, Ntumy & Tweneboah, 2005; Aniteye, 2002; Lassey, 1995; Obed & Wilson, 1999). In the two main teaching hospitals in Ghana, Korle Bu and Komfo Anokye, Teaching Hospitals, abortion complications constitute about 50% of gynaecological admissions (Aniteye, 2002; Turpin, Danso & Odoi, 2000). The commonest reason why women sought an abortion was not having the financial means to take care of a child. Other reasons reported included wanting to delay childbearing or complete school. The Ghana Maternal Health Survey (GMHS, 2007) which took place almost a decade after Ahiadeke's study (1997/98) showed some similar findings; most women having abortions are young and women seek abortion services from both orthodox and traditional sources. It appears relatively more women sought help from a doctor in the nationally representative survey than in the study that concentrated in southern Ghana. This may be due to a growing awareness of the need for safe abortion although the continuing high level of maternal mortality in Ghana suggests that access to safe abortion is still constrained.

Preventing Unsafe Abortions

Unsafe abortions and their deleterious effects are preventable via primary, secondary and tertiary preventive initiatives (Okonofua, 2004). Primary prevention focuses largely on effective contraception including emergency contraception to avert unwanted pregnancies, the main cause of unsafe abortion. Pragmatic health education programmes with an emphasis on human sexuality, reproductive and sexual health matters among adolescents, the marginalized and vulnerable populations are important. They will help such people make informed choices about their sexuality to help compensate for the unmet needs for family planning among them. Secondary prevention of unsafe abortion involves the provision of safe abortion within the framework of the existing laws. However, African countries are reportedly characterized by restrictive laws which render access to safe abortion services difficult. In Nigeria, for example, the law criminalizes abortion unless the pregnancy threatens the woman's life. Due to these legal restrictions, religious and social norms that prohibit abortion and the social stigma associated with abortion in Nigeria, its practice is shrouded in secrecy; many unskilled providers perform abortions clandestinely often in dangerous and unhygienic settings (Makinwa-Adebusaye, Singh, & Audam, 1997).

Okonofua (2004) highlights how legal restrictions lead to underground abortion practices that severely compromise the safety of the woman. Abortion is also restricted in Kenya and safe abortion is only accessible to wealthy women, an indication of gross health inequity. Maternal mortality in Kenya is very high at about 590 deaths per 100,000 live births (similar to that of Ghana) of which about 30 percent are attributable to unsafe abortion (Brookman-Amissah & Moyo, 2004). A national assessment of the magnitude and consequences of unsafe abortion in Kenya in 2003 showed that more than 300,000 women have unsafe abortions every year. Also more than 20,000 women suffer from complications of unsafe abortion yearly; among them, an estimated 2,000 women die. There are public debates and proposals to liberalize the law (Brookman-Amissah & Moyo, 2004).

A few countries such as South Africa and Tunisia allow women with unwanted pregnancy to have abortion on demand. However, in countries such as Ghana and Zambia, even though the abortion laws are liberal, women have difficulty accessing safe abortion services due to socio-cultural and service-related barriers. The liberality of Zambia's abortion law lies in the fact that it allows abortions to be carried out on broad health as well as socio-economic grounds. The law also permits abortion where continuation of the pregnancy would involve risk to the life or injury to the physical or mental health of the pregnant woman or any existing children of the pregnant woman. Although Zambia's maternal mortality ratio has declined since abortion was legalised, from 729/100,000 live births in 2001 to 591/100,000 live births as of 2007, the reduction is considered insignificant (Mbewe, 2010). Barriers to safe abortion still exist in Zambia. For example, restrictive administrative policies still render abortion services inaccessible (Berer, 2002; Whitaker & Germain, 1999). Three doctors are required to approve a woman's request for an abortion. This is a very difficult requirement to meet given the scarcity of doctors, especially in rural areas. Other barriers to service provision in Zambia are reluctant providers, lack of trained providers and other resources and failure to authorize providers and facilities (Berer, 2002). Okonofua (2004) reiterates that despite these liberal legal provisions, women still have limited access to safe abortion due to an array of socio-cultural and service-related barriers. In the case of Ghana, which also has a relatively liberal law in the sense that it allows abortion to preserve 'physical and mental health', it is puzzling that there has been little impact on the maternal mortality ratio since the law was introduced in 1985. This suggests that while having a liberal law in place is important, and a necessary first step, a lot also depends on how that law is interpreted and implemented.

Legal Interpretation and Implementation

In some cases, laws may be very similar on paper, but interpreted and applied differently in practice (e.g. Britain and Ghana). Abortion laws differ from country to country according to the way in which they are formulated within national legislation (United Nations 2001a, 2001b, 2002). Abortion may be captured in the criminal code, in civil law, public health codes or medical ethics codes. In Ghana it appears in the criminal code. In some countries, these documents clearly show how abortion laws should be interpreted. However, in many countries there are no guidelines for interpretation. This omission may give rise to problems with implementation. Also, in countries where the laws and policies have many ambiguous clauses, this lack of clarity makes the law difficult to comprehend, resulting in problems of interpretation and implementation. Cook and Dickens (2003) also observe that in countries with restrictive laws, there are hardly any guidelines for interpreting clauses that are not explicit but prone to multiple interpretation as in the definition of the concept of 'risk'. This lack of clarity in their view makes health providers brand all abortions illegal and then provide it in secrecy. Furthermore, Whitaker and Germain (1999) consider abortion laws as difficult to interpret and frequently unknown to women and health providers, hence restricting access to legal abortion in most African countries. All these factors affect the availability of, and women's access to, safe, legal abortion services (WHO, 2003) and decriminalizing the law must be accompanied by measures to facilitate its implementation (Hessini, 2005).

In addition to the legal and policy-related factors that pose challenges to the provision of safe abortion services, there is ample evidence that other service-related and socio-cultural factors impinge on abortion provision even within the framework of the law. Many studies have demonstrated that across a range of countries, women who require safe abortion services that are legal are not able to access them for reasons such as paucity of approved facilities, inadequacy of trained providers who are willing to provide the service, poor quality of services, and long waiting times (delays) are also common (Althaus, 2000; Benson, 2005; Berer, 2002; Dickson, 2003; Duggal & Ramachandran, 2004; Garcia, 2004; Gupte, Bandewar & Pisal, 1997; Harries, Orner, Gabriel & Mitchell, 2007; Henshaw 1998; Iyengar & Iyengar, 2002; Koster-Oyekan 1998; Prada 2005; United Nations, 2001a, 2001b, 2002; Warriner, Duolao Wang, My Huong, 2011). Health providers' attitudes emerged as a major influence to access. In general, the service-related barriers relate to legal and policy ambiguities and inconsistencies, provider attitudes and lack of training while important socio-cultural barriers include cultural values, social norms, and moral and religious objections which create dilemmas in professional practice. After the multiplicity of factors that influence secondary prevention of unsafe abortion, the third preventive measure is discussed below.

Tertiary prevention of unsafe abortion is about providing post-abortion care. This includes post-abortion contraceptives as an integral component for the prevention of recurrent abortions. Post-abortion care has been the main strategy to reduce abortion-related mortality in Africa (Hord & Wolf, 2004). It comprises the management of abortion complications using inexpensive technology such as Manual Vacuum Aspiration, effective counselling of women who have had an abortion and provision of effective post-abortion contraceptives (Okonofua, 2004).

The Advent of Comprehensive Abortion Care (CAC)

Generally, public discussions on abortion and its legality are rare but at the 1994 International Conference on Population and Development (ICPD) held in Cairo and the 1995 Fourth World Conference on Women held in Beijing, abortion was discussed at length (Crane & Hord Smith 2006; Rosoff, 1999). These two conferences are important for a number of reasons. They created awareness among nations, and initiated global discussion on the burden of unsafe abortion and the need for action. Furthermore, the ICPD included safe abortion services as a reproductive right in countries where they were legal and post-abortion care as a reproductive right in countries where abortion per se was not legal, creating obligations for governments that signed the declaration. The Programme of Action of the ICPD (1994) was the first major international agreement to make recommendations on unsafe abortion (Hessini, 2005). The meeting called govern-ments' attention to the public health impact of unsafe abortion and the urgent need to reduce recourse to abortion by expanding contraceptive services. Women with unwanted pregnancies were to be offered reliable information, compassionate counselling and safe abortion services where abortion is not against the law. In addition, the meeting required that women have access to quality services for the management of complications of unsafe abortion coupled with post-abortion counselling, education and family planning services to prevent recurrent abortions (Hessini, 2005).

In response to the Programme of Action from the International Conference on Population and Development (ICPD), the Platform for Action of the Fourth World Conference on Women in Beijing, the ICPD+5 Meeting and other international consensus meetings such as the Conference of African Union Ministers of Health and the African

Regional Conference on Unsafe Abortion, governments were called upon to show commitment to addressing the problem by ensuring access to safe abortion within the framework of national laws (AGI, 1999; Faundes, Duarte, Neto & De Sousa, 2004; Gerhardt, 1997; Hessini et al., 2006; Sai, 2002). To facilitate this task, the World Health Organization (WHO, 2003) developed norms and standards for providing quality abortion services entitled: '*Safe Abortion: Technical and Policy Guidance for Health Systems*'. Drawing on this guidance, countries have instituted pragmatic strategies and interventions geared towards combating unsafe abortions and ensuring that women's rights to reproductive health are realized (Hessini et al., 2006).

Ghana is one such country. Ghana has taken a number of steps to reduce maternal mortality attributable to unsafe abortions. These steps date back to 1985 when the former law on abortion was liberalized to become PNDC Law 102 which allows abortion in the following instances:

i) Where the continuation of the pregnancy would involve risk to the life of the pregnant mother or injury to her physical or mental health;

ii) Where there is a substantial risk that if the child is born it may suffer from or later develop a serious physical abnormality or disease;

iii) Where the pregnancy is the result of rape, defilement of a female idiot or incest.

In the West African sub-region, Ghana is noted as the country with an abortion law that is relatively liberal; however, even though the law permits abortion on broad grounds including physical and mental health, there is limited access to safe, legal abortion services. This is due in part to the lack of policies translating the law into services, which is also influenced by the lack of clarity in the law (Aboagye et al., 2007; Lithur, 2004; Morhee & Morhee, 2006). In a review of the National Reproductive Health Policy and Standards document in 2003, there was an addition of the objective '*to provide abortion care services as permitted by law*'. This was captured under the section: '*Prevention and management of unsafe abortion and post-abortion care*'.

The need therefore arose for safe abortion services to be provided to the extent permitted by the law (GHS, 2003).

The Road Map to Comprehensive Abortion Care (Safe Abortion Services and Post-Abortion Care)

In March 2003, IPAS – International Pregnancy Advisory Services organized a meeting in Addis Ababa, Ethiopia, on 'Action to reduce maternal mortality in Africa' (Hessini et al., 2006). At this meeting, the WHO (2003) publication, 'Safe abortion: technical and policy guidance for health systems', which discussed how countries could ensure access to safe abortion services to the extent permitted by law, was discussed and adopted by countries represented. Ghana sent Ministry of Health (MOH) representatives to this meeting. Following the meeting, a communiqué was signed by all the countries that were represented (Hessini et al., 2006). Each country decided to take action to reduce maternal mortality. After that, Ghana formed a group of people from various disciplines related to reproductive health to make sure the recommendations of the meeting were put in action. The Ghana Health Service (GHS), having been charged with the mandate of reducing the high levels of maternal mortality, formed a taskforce whose duty was to come up with a strategic plan to address the problem of unsafe abortion in Ghana. In December 2003, the plan was adopted by key stakeholders. In order to further reduce the toll of maternal deaths attributable to unsafe abortions, the GHS revised the National Reproductive Health Service Policy and Standards (GHS, 2003) incorporating the additional objective noted above to allow for provision of safe abortion services to the full extent of the law.

In May/June 2005, a strategic assessment of abortion and abortion care services was carried out under the leadership of the GHS and an advisory committee of policy makers (GHS 2005). The purpose of the assessment was to enable key stakeholders to hold discussions with various communities in the country on issues of interest in reproductive health, including unwanted pregnancy, contraception and abortion. Measures to reduce abortion–related deaths and how to improve access to and quality of care in abortion services to the full extent of the law were also to be explored. The assessment was done by a team comprising 17 stakeholders, some of whom were policy makers, programme managers, service providers, reproductive rights activists and women's health advocates. It covered the Upper East, Northern, Brong Ahafo, Ashanti, Greater Accra and Central regions of Ghana. The major findings included the poor knowledge of the abortion law among the public and even health providers and the dangerous methods used by women and girls for induced abortion. Other findings were the strong *'culture of silence'* that surrounded abortion and related issues and the current willingness of communities to openly discuss abortion issues. In addition, the high cost of abortion services and the clandestine nature in which these services were provided were also discussed. It was established that women and girls in the study area had a high unmet need for contraception. The upsurge of medical abortion in urban areas was another significant finding during the assessment (GHS, 2005). Based on these important findings and in response to the expanded objectives in the GHS 2003 RH policy to provide abortion services to the extent permitted by law, the Standards and Protocols for the Prevention and Management of Unsafe Abortion were developed in 2006 to provide technical and managerial guidance for the provision of comprehensive abortion care services of desired quality (GHS, 2006). The development of the standards and protocols was in fulfillment of a commitment on the part of the international community to address the problem of unsafe abortion partially through the provision of safe abortion (UN, ICPD Report, 1994). It was in response to a call by WHO on health systems to ensure the availability of safe abortion services in accordance with national laws and supported by policies, regulations and health systems infrastructure (WHO, 2003).

Following these developments, periodic meetings were held by key stakeholders, and doctors and midwives who did not object to the provision of safe abortion services were trained. Based on some selected communities' response (during the strategic assessment) to the provision of comprehensive abortion care in public health facilities, these services have currently been initiated in some public facilities in the country. Abortion services, within the confines of the law, are now being provided in some Ghanaian public health facilities by trained doctors and midwives who are not conscientious objectors. Although comprehensive abortion care (which includes safe abortion services and post abortion care) are currently being provided in reproductive and child health units of some of our public health institutions, there are on-going heated debates about health and moral issues concerning the provision of abortion services in public health facilities in Ghana.

The provision of safe, legal abortions and women's access to safe abortion services is a highly contested issue globally, involving moral, religious, ethical, and medical debates that could be unending. The debates centre on women's autonomy and their right to decide whether to keep an unplanned pregnancy or terminate it. The other side of the debate is whether the foetus is a person with rights, quite simply the right to live.

A recent policy-oriented qualitative study in Ghana (Aniteye, 2012) which looked at why safe abortion services are not provided in public health facilities despite a liberal legal framework, identified some important areas of argument both for and against abortion. In this study, a sample of 76 key stakeholders were purposively selected from three (3) hospitals, five (5) urban health centres and two (2) health-related NGOs in Accra and interviewed. Most of the key stakeholders who took part in the study including health professionals (obstetrician/gynaecologists, midwives and pharmacists), non-health professionals (legal practitioners, parliamentarians, policy makers and researchers) and religious leaders, outlined arguments based on 'public health', 'professional ethics' and 'human rights issues' giving reasons on one hand why abortion services should be provided for women who need it. On the other hand, arguments mainly based on morality, religion and the rights of the foetus were advanced against provision of safe abortion services for women who had pregnancies they called unwanted.

In relation to public health, the proponents of safe abortion in the study argued for provision of safe abortion services within the national legal framework, given the many lives that are lost needlessly due to abortions provided clandestinely by untrained persons under unhygienic conditions. In addition to the deaths of women from unsafe abortions, there were references to women who are maimed from complications of abortions. Reducing maternal morbidity and mortality resulting from unsafe abortions was deemed a crucial public health imperative. Among the health professionals interviewed in the study, some thought that irrespective of their religious inclinations and beliefs, they were obliged by their mandate as health professionals to safeguard women's health and life by providing abortion services for women who needed them. This, they referred to as "professional ethics". Some obstetricians and policy makers (who were medical doctors now working at the MOH) referred to the *Hippocratic Oath* they had sworn as the basis for their actions. Ironically, this Oath forbids abortion but calls on medical practitioners to save lives and do no harm. Interestingly, some midwives also referred to the *Midwives' Prayer* as their mandate to preserve life, which in this instance is the life of the foetus. Thus, while obstetricians were largely in favour of saving women's lives, midwives were highly conservative about the provision of safe abortions. While the attitudes of the obstetricians, policy makers and pharmacists were due to exposure to training and work outside Ghana, as well as knowledge of the abortion law, international conventions and treaties; in contrast the midwives' attitudes were largely informed by their religious beliefs and less exposure to work and training outside Ghana and a lack of knowledge of the abortion law, international treaties and conventions. Lastly, based on Ghana's ratification of international treaties on human rights, a significant number of stakeholders, mainly obstetricians and policy makers, posited that women who request abortion services ought to have access to such services within the framework of the national law.

On the other side of the abortion divide, some stakeholders — mainly midwives, religious leaders and an obstetrician — argued strongly against abortion. They said the procedure is morally wrong and unethical, that the foetus is a person and has rights which are being violated. One major source of argument against the practice of abortion was religious beliefs which, by inference, equate abortion with murder, an act forbidden by both Christianity and Islam. A number of Biblical passages were cited as being against the practice of abortion, the most popular being Jeremiah 1:4-5 and Psalm 139:

13-16; others included Luke 1:15; Genesis 25:21–23 and Matthew 1:18. There were some dissenting views among the key stakeholders. Even though the vast majority of midwives were against the provision of abortion in public health facilities, a few thought the procedure was sometimes necessary. One obstetrician spoke vehemently against abortion; he was Catholic by religion. Two religious leaders, a hospital Chaplain and a Moslem Cleric (who was a pharmacy technologist) were in favour of abortion because of their experiences with abortion cases in their workplace.

Conclusion

In conclusion, unsafe abortion is a public health problem that warrants global action by committed governments. Global and local estimates of the magnitude of the burden of unsafe abortion are colossal yet the problem is largely preventable. The three levels of prevention can help mitigate the effects of unsafe abortion on families, communities and the nation. Given that the contraceptive prevalence rate in Ghana is low (GDHS, 2003) and that only a quarter of currently married women are using a method of contraception, that 34 percent of currently married women have unmet need for family planning, and 40 percent of all pregnancies are unwanted or mistimed, the importance of family planning as a primary preventive measure cannot be overemphasized. Primary prevention requires effective family planning thus the obvious need for family planning to be repositioned and revamped to increase its use by the population. In relation to unsafe abortion, secondary prevention involves the provision of safe abortion services within national legal frameworks. The need for provision of safe abortion services has been reiterated by ICPD and other international conventions and treaties. It is argued that there should be access to safe abortion services where the procedure is allowed by law. Where women have had recourse to abortion with the attending complications, post-abortion care (PAC), a tertiary preventive measure should be accessible to these women to safeguard their health and lives. The provision of post-abortion care to women with abortion complications constitutes tertiary prevention.

Hitherto, abortion services have not been openly available in public health facilities in Ghana. Since 1985, Ghana's abortion law permits abortion for cases of rape, incest, foetal abnormality and where the woman's physical and mental health would be affected when the pregnancy is kept. Stakeholders' debates concerning availability of safe abortion in public health facilities border on public health issues, professional ethics and the rights of women; these arguments are advanced for the services. On the other hand, religious and moral arguments backed by biblical verses have been advanced against abortion. Following international consensus meetings and Ghana's ratification of treaties, safe abortion services are now available in public health facilities through the efforts of some key stakeholders in reproductive health. There appear to be three overriding issues regarding access to safe abortion services. First, legality of abortion appears to affect availability and use of safe services. Secondly, services and resources available (infrastructure, equipment and training) are important for ensuring legal services are in fact provided. Thirdly, social acceptability and social access issues – related especially to religion and morality – are critical influences on whether potential clients are willing and able to use available services.

References

Aboagye, B., & Akosa, A.B. (2000). An autopsy study of maternal deaths. *Ghana Medical Journal, 34,* (3): 152-156.

Aboagye, P. K., Gebreselassie, H., Quansah Asare, G., Mitchell, E.M.H. & Addy, J. (2007). An assessment of the readiness to offer contraceptives and comprehensive abortion care in the Greater Accra, Eastern and Ashanti regions of Ghana. Chapel Hill: Ipas.

Adanu, R.M., Ntumy, M.N., & Tweneboah, E. (2005). Profile of women with abortion complications in Ghana. *Trop Doct. 35*(3):139-42.

Ahiadeke, C. (2001). Incidence of Induced Abortion in southern Ghana. *International Family Planning Perspectives, 27,*(2): 96-101.

Ahman, E., & Shah, I. (2004). Unsafe Abortion Global and Regional Estimates of the Incidence of Unsafe Abortion and Associated Mortality in 2000. 4th ed. Geneva: WHO.

Alan Guttmacher Institute. (1999). *Sharing Responsibility : Women, Society and Abortion Worldwide*. New York: Alan Guttmacher Institute.

Althaus, F. A. (2000). Work in Progress: The Expansion of Access to Abortion Services in South Africa Following Legalization. *International Family Planning Perspectives, 26,* 84-86.

Aniteye, P. (2002). Reasons, Methods and Health Outcomes of Induced Abortion: A Study of Women on Admission with Abortion Complications. (Unpublished) MPhil.Thesis. University of Ghana.

Baird, T.L., Billings, D.L. & Demuyakor, B. (2000). Community education efforts enhance post-abortion care programs in Ghana. *Am J Public Health, 90,*(40): 631-2.

Benson, J. (2005). Evaluating Abortion-Care Programs: Old Challenges, New Directions. *Studies in Family Planning, 36,* (3): 189-202.

Berer, M. (2002). Making Abortions Safe: A Matter of Good Public Health Policy and Practice. *Reproductive Health Matters, 10* (19): 31-44.

Braam, T., & Hessini, L. (2004). The Power Dynamics Perpetuating Unsafe Abortion in Africa: A Feminist Perspective. *African Journal of Reproductive Health, 8,* (1): 43-51.

Brookman-Amissah, E., & Moyo, J.B. (2004). Abortion Law Reform in Sub-Saharan Africa: No Turning Back. *Reproductive Health Matters, 12,* (24): 227-234.

Cook, R.J., & Dickens, B.M. (2003). Human rights dynamics of abortion law reform. *Human Rights Quarterly, 25,*(1):1-59.

Crane, B.B., & Hord Smith, C.E. (2006). Access to safe abortion: An Essential Strategy for Achieving the Millennium Development Goals to Improve Maternal Health, Promote Gender Equality, and Reduce Poverty. Background paper to: Bernstein, S. and Hanson, C.J. Public Choices, Private Decisions: Sexual and Reproductive Health and the Millennium Development Goals. New York: UN Millennium Project.

Dickson, K.A. (2003). Freedom of Religion and the Church. Accra: Ghana Universities Press.

Duggal, R. & Ramachandran, V. (2004). The Abortion Assessment Project: India — Key Findings and Recommendations. *Reproductive Health Matters, 12* (24 Supp): 122-129.

Faundes, A., Duarte, G.A., Neto, J.A. & De Sousa, M.H., (2004). The closer you are, the better you understand: the reaction of Brazillian obstetrician/gynaecologists to unwanted pregnancy. *Reproductive Health Matters,12,* (24): 47-56.

Garcia, S.G., Tatum, C., Becker, D. et al. (2004). Policy implications of a national opinion survey on abortion in Mexico. *Reproductive Health Matters, 12,* (24): 65-74.

Geelhoed, D.W., Visser, L.E., Asare, K., Schagen van Leeuwen, J.H., & van Roosmalen, J. (2003). Trends in maternal mortality: a 13-year hospital-based study in rural Ghana. *Eur J Obstet Gynecol Reprod Biol, 107,* (2): 135-9.

Gerhardt, A.J. (1997). Abortion laws into action: implementing legal reform. *Initiat Reprod Health Policy, 2,* (1): 1-3.

Ghana Health Service. (2006). *Prevention and Management of Unsafe Abortion: Comprehensive Abortion Care Services. Standards and Protocols.* Accra.

Ghana Health Service (2005). *A Strategic Assessment of Comprehensive Abortion Care in Ghana. Report.*

Ghana Health Service (2003). *National Reproductive Health Service Policy and Standards.* 2nd ed. Accra: GHS.

Ghana Statistical Service (GSS), Ghana Health Service (GHS), and Macro International. (2009). *Ghana Maternal Health Survey,* 2007. Calverton: GSS, GHS, and Macro International.

Gupte, M., Bandewar, S., & Pisal, H. (1997). Abortion needs of women in India: a case study of rural Maharashtra. *Reproductive Health Matters, 5,* (9):77-86.

Harries, J., Orner, P., Gabriel, M., & Mitchell, E. (2007). Delays in seeking an abortion until the second trimester: a qualitative study in South Africa. *Reprod Health,* 4:7.

Hessini, L. (2005). Global Progress in Abortion Advocacy and Policy: An Assessment of the Decade since ICPD. *Reproductive Health Matters, 13,* (25):88-100.

Hessini, L., Brookman-Amissah, E., & Crane, B.B. (2006). Global policy change and women's access to safe abortion: The impact of the World Health Organization's guidance in Africa. *Afr J Reprod Health, 10,* (3):14-27.

Hord, C., & Wolf, M. (2004). Breaking the Cycle of Unsafe Abortion in Africa. *African Journal of Reproductive Health, 8,* (1): 29-36.

Iyengar, K., & Iyengar, S.D. (2002). Elective abortion as a primary health service in rural India: experience with manual vacuum aspiration. *Reproductive Health Matters,* 10 (19): 55-64.

Koster-Oyekan, (1998). Cited in safe abortion: Technical and policy guidance for health systems. Geneva: WHO. (2003; p. 84).

Lassey, A.T. (1995). Complications of induced abortions and their prevention in Ghana. *East African Medical Journal, 72,* (12):774-777.

Lithur, N.O. (2005). Safe abortion is legally permissible — declares ex-FIDA boss. *The Ghanaian Chronicle,15,* (28) 10 October 2005.

Lithur, N.O. (2004). Destigmatising Abortion: Expanding Community Awareness of Abortion as a Reproductive Health Issue in Ghana. *African Journal of Reproductive Health, 8,* (1): 70-74.

Makinwa-Adebusaye, P., Singh S., & Audam, S. (1997). Nigerian Health Professionals Perception about Abortion Practice. *Int Fam Plan Persp,* 23:155-161.

Makinwa-Adebusoye, P. (1992). Sexual behaviours, reproductive knowledge and contraceptive use among urban Nigerians. *Int Fam Plan Persp. 18,* (2): 66-70.

Mayhew, S. (2004).Sexual and Reproductive Health in Ghana and the Role of Donor Assistance. A Case study. www.populationaction.or/Publica-tions/Reports/Progress_andPromises/asset_upload_file36_5855.pdf.

Mbewe, R. (2010). MOH reviewing law on abortion. Available at: http://www.postzambia.com/post-read_article.php?articleId=10248.
[Accessed on 3 June 2011].

Ministry of Health (2008). National Consultative Meeting on the Reduction of Maternal Mortality in Ghana: Partnership for Action. A Synthesis Report. Accra: Ministry of Health.

Ministry of Health/Ghana Health Service. (2005). *An assessment of the provision of comprehensive abortion care to the full extent of the law.* Supported by Ipas with the technical assistance of the World Health Organization. Accra: MoH/GHS.

Ministry of Health and Ghana Statistical Service. (2003). *Ghana Demographic and Health Survey* 2003. Accra: MOH/GSS.

Ministry of Health (1996). *National Reproductive Health Service Policy and Standards.* Accra: Ministry of Health.

Morhee, E.S.K., Morhee, R.A.S., & Danso, K.A. (2007). Attitudes of doctors toward establishing safe abortion units in Ghana. *International Journal of Gynaecology and Obstetrics, 98,*70-74.

Morhee, R.A.S., and Morhee, E.S.K. (2006). Overview of the Law and Availa-bility of Abortion Services in Ghana. *Ghana Med J 40(3): 80-86.*

Mundigo, A. L., and Indriso, C. (1999). *Abortion in the Developing World.* New Dehli: Vistaar Publications.

National Population Council. (2000). Adolescent Reproductive Health Policy. Accra: Harris Standard Graphics.

Nursing and Midwifery Council, Ghana. *Code of Ethics.* Available at: http://www.nmcgh.org/ethic.html.

Ngwena C. (2004). An appraisal of abortion laws in southern Africa from a reproductive health rights perspective. Journal of Law, Medicine and Ethics. 32(4); 708-717.

Obed, S.A., & Wilson, J.B. (1999). Uterine perforation from induced abortion at KorleBu Teaching Hospital, Accra, Ghana: A five-year review. *WAJM.* Vol. 18 No 4. Oct-Dec.

Okonofua, F. (2004). Breaking the Silence on Prevention of Unsafe Abortion in *Africa. Afr. J Reprod Health 8 (1):7-10.*

Prada, E. et al. (2005). Abortion and Post-Abortion Care in Guatemala: A Report from Health Care Professionals and Health Facilities. Occasional Report No. 18. New York: Guttmacher Institute.

Ravindran, J. (2003).Unwanted pregnancy - medical and ethical dimensions. *Med J Malaysia.* Mar; 58 Suppl A:23-35.

Rossof, J. (1999). *Sharing Responsibility: Women, Society and Abortion Worldwide.* New York: Guttmacher Institute.

Sai, F. (2002). *Fred Sai speaks out.* Revised edition. London: IPPF.

Sedgh, G., Singh, S., Henshaw, S.K., & Bankole, A. (2007). Induced abortion: estimated rates and trends worldwide. *The Lancet 370(9595) 1338-1345.*

Sedgh, G., Singh, S., Henshaw, S.K. & Bankole, A. (2012). Induced abortion: incidence and trends worldwide from 1995 to 2008. *The Lancet 379* (9816) 625-632.

The Criminal Code (Amendment) Law, (1985). PNDC L 102. Accra and Tema: The Gazette. Ghana Publishing Corporation.

Turpin, C.A., Danso, K.A., & Odoi, A.T. (2000). Abortion at Komfo Anokye Teaching Hospital. *Ghana Medical Journal. 36 (2): 60-64.*

United Nations. (1994). Programme of Action adopted at the International Conference on Population and Development, (ICPD) Cairo. Available at: http://www.un.org/popin/icpd/conference/offeng/poa.html.

United Nations. (2001). Abortion policies: a global review. Volume 1: Afghanistan to France. New York: United Nations. (ST/ESA/SER.A/187).

United Nations (2001b). Abortion policies; a global review. Volume 2. Gabon to Norway. New York: United Nations. (ST/ESA/SER.A/191).

United Nations. (2002). Abortion policies: a global review. Volume 3 Oman to Zimbabwe. New York, United Nations. (ST/ESA/SER.A/196).

Warriner, I.K. et al. (2011). Can mid-level healthcare providers administer early medical abortion as safely and effectively as doctors? A randomised controlled equivalence trial in Nepal. *The Lancet*. Volume 377, Issue 9772. 1155-1161.

Whitaker, C. and Germain, A. (1999). Safe Abortion in Africa: Ending the Silence and Starting a Movement. *African Journal of Reproductive Health* 3 (2):7-14.

World Health Organization. (2012). Safe abortion: technical and policy guidance for health systems. 2nd ed. Geneva: WHO.

World Health Organization. (2011). Unsafe Abortion: global and regional estimates of the incidence of unsafe abortion and associated mortality in 2008, 6th ed. Geneva: WHO.

World Health Organization. (2004). Maternal Mortality in 2000: Estimates developed by WHO, UNICEF and UNFPA. Geneva: WHO.

World Health Organization. (2003). Safe Abortion: Technical and Policy Guidance for Health Systems. Geneva: WHO. p. 98.

World Health Organization. (2002). *The World Health Report*. Geneva: WHO.

World Health Organization. (1998). Unsafe Abortion: Global and Regional Estimates of Incidence of and Mortality Due to Abortion, with a listing of Available Country Data. 3rd ed. Geneva: WHO.

Zambia's Abortion Law. Available at: http://www.un.org/esa/population/publications/abortion/doc/zambia/.doc. [Accessed on: 22 August 2009].

Chapter Ten

Trends in the Management of Diabetes Mellitus: Nurses' Perspectives

Kwadwo Ameyaw Korsah

Introduction

Nurses play crucial roles in the management of diabetic patients in healthcare settings. It is therefore very important for nurses to be familiar with the trends in the management of diabetes mellitus. Apart from the medical management of diabetics, nurses need to know the socio-cultural issues surrounding diabetes as part of the current trend in the management of the condition. Improved knowledge of the issues relating to the condition among nurses will translate into enhanced management of the condition, preventing complications and leading to overall improvement in the quality of life of diabetic patients. As part of the current trend in the management of the condition, the totality of patient is paramount, which goes beyond the identification of clinical manifestations and commencement of a medical regimen by nurses and other providers.

Diabetes mellitus (DM) is a chronic, non-communicable disease and also one of the major global public health issues. It produces many complex changes and poses significant socioeconomic challenges for individuals who are affected (Mbaya et al., 2010). The International Diabetes Federation (IDF) estimated in 2009 that the worldwide number of adults with diabetes will increase by 54 percent, from 284.6 million in 2010 to 438.4 million in 2030 (International Diabetes Federation, 2009). Diabetes is diagnosed if the Fasting Blood Sugar (FBS) value is more than or equal to 5.7 mmol/l (102.6mg/dl), or if the Random Blood Sugar value is more than or equal to 7.8mmol/l (140.4mg/dl), or if the Plasma Glucose value two hours after a 75g oral load of glucose is greater than or equal to 11.1 mmol/l (200mg/dl) (Standard Treatment Guidelines for Ghana, 2010). The Oral Glucose Tolerance Test (OGTT) is ordered as a gold standard method to confirm the condition. In this test, the patient is asked to fast for eight to twelve hours before the test is performed. Then, a 75g oral load of glucose solution is given to the patient and blood value of glucose is checked after two hours. Diabetes mellitus is confirmed if the blood glucose level is 11.1mmol/l (200mg/dl) after the two-hour period (Expert Committee, 1997). In asymptomatic individuals, performing the Fasting Blood Sugar (FBS) test on one occasion is not enough to establish the diagnosis (i.e. basis to treat).

Classification of Diabetes Mellitus

Classification of diabetes mellitus is based on the 1997 Expert Committee's report under the auspices of the World Health Organization and the American Diabetes Association which categorized diabetes mellitus in four main groups. These are Type 1, Type 2, "other specific types" and gestational diabetes (Expert Committee, 2003). This classification by the experts for diabetes mellitus was based on aetiology.

Diabetes Type 1 is characterised by beta cell destruction caused by an autoimmune reaction, usually leading to absolute insulin deficiency in which an external source of insulin is required for survival by the affected individual. It is also known that individuals with human leukocyte antigen (HLA), which is used in tissue typing, develop diabetes Type 1. This issue has been contested on the grounds that some individuals develop diabetes but they do not possess the HLA (Fain, 1998). The onset of this type of diabetes is usually acute, with signs developing over a period of a few days to weeks. It has been noted that over 95 percent of persons with diabetes Type 1 develop the disease before the age of 25, with an equal incidence in both sexes and an increased prevalence in the white population (Expert Committee, 2003).

Type 2 diabetes mellitus is caused by lifestyle factors in association with genetic factors. It forms about 90 percent of all diabetes cases. In other words, the aetiology of diabetes Type 2 is multi-factorial with a considerable genetic component but the disease is lifestyle and environment-related (Expert Committee, 2003). The predisposing factors for type 2 diabetes mellitus are obesity, physical inactivity, hypertension, hyperlidaemia, sedentary lifestyle, and intake of fatty foods, which are all associated with urbanization and modernization (Zimmet, 2000), as well as aging. Although, Type 2 diabetes is mainly a condition of adults, current research investigations show that there is increasing prevalence in adolescents and children as well (Reinehr & Wabitisch, 2005). It has been observed that the rapid rise of childhood obesity and its association with the development of diabetes has led to anticipation that Type 2 diabetes has the potential to result in a decline in the overall life expectancy of the global population within the first half of this century (Olshansky, Passera & Hershow, 2005).

Diabetes categorised as "other specific types" is associated with genetic defects of beta cell activities which include diseases associated with exocrine pancreas such as pancreatitis, and dysfunction linked to other endocrinopathies, for example, pancreatic dysfunction caused by drugs, chemicals or infection and other similar factors (Expert Committee, 2003).

Pregnancy-induced diabetes mellitus is termed Gestational Diabetes Mellitus (GDM). This categorization affects women in whom the condition is identified during the pregnancy period but the disease resolves after delivery. These individuals are at increased risk of developing diabetes Type 1 or 2 later in life, but with a high possibility of developing Type 2 diabetes mellitus. After pregnancy, diagnostic classification may be changed to Insulin Dependent Diabetes Mellitus (IDDM) or Non-Insulin Dependent Diabetes Mellitus (NIDDM). Women who had the disease before the pregnancy are not included in this classification. In pregnancy, a lot of hormones and other chemicals are produced, most of which are antagonistic to insulin production (Jonanovic & Pettitt, 2001). This means in pregnancy, insulin requirement goes up due to the phenomenon of increasing manufacture of insulin inhibitors or antagonists. Examples of insulin antagonists are human placental lactogen, placental insulinase, cortisol, oestrogens and progesterone The increased production of insulin antagonists in many cases happens during the last three months of pregnancy (American Diabetes Association, 2004).

Clinical Manifestations of Diabetes Mellitus

When diagnosed, individuals have four cardinal clinical manifestations (Fain, 1998). These are:

1. Extreme weight loss and muscular wasting due to breakdown of protein and lipids (catabolism).
2. Frequent urination (polyuria) because glucose attracts water and an osmotic diuresis occurs. This polyuria results in the loss of water and electrolytes, particularly Sodium (Na), Chloride (Cl), Potassium (K) and Phosphate (Ph). If the concentration of glucose in the blood is sufficiently high, the kidney may not reabsorb all of the filtered glucose; the glucose then appears in urine (Glucosuria). Fluid loss through the kidneys results as the kidneys work to excrete the increased load of glucose, producing loss of water, sodium (Na), magnesium, calcium, potassium chloride, and phosphate.
3. Excessive thirst (polydypsia): The loss of water and sodium results in thirst and increases fluid intake.
4. Excessive eating (polyphagia): Extreme hunger and increased food intake are triggered as the cells become starved of their fuel. Other manifestations are weakness, and blurred vision (Fain, 1998).

Psychological Manifestations of Diabetes Mellitus

The onset of diabetes mellitus leads to psychological manifestations in addition to the physical manifestations already mentioned. These may include mild depression, anxiety, anger, and somatic complaints at the time of diagnosis. These symptoms are usually temporary and resolve within 6 to 9 months. However, in some patients the depressive and anxiety symptoms may continue to increase within the duration of diabetes (Schiffrin, 2001). Research studies have shown that some parents displace their frustrations, anxiety and anger on their children who are diagnosed with diabetes, probably due to perceived burden their child's condition places on them (Schiffrin, 2001). Other psychological manifestations of diabetes mellitus reported in the literature are apprehension and fear of complications of eyesight, illness or pain related to diabetes, tiredness or lack of energy, fear of moving from tablet medications unto insulin injections and fear of their condition getting worse (Woodcock & Kinmonth, 2001).

Management of Diabetes Mellitus

As part of diabetes management, it is always important to take a thorough history from the patient about the condition. As already noted above, the patient may complain of polyuria, polydipsia, polyphagia and weight loss. The severity of these manifestations will inform the nurse of the nature of the patient's problem. The patient may be asymptomatic, which means that the cardinal manifestations mentioned above may be incidental findings. It is also likely that affected individuals may present with complications such as purititis vulvae or balanitis, mental apathy, confusion, retinopathy, neuropathy, nephropathy, infections, hyperlipidaemia and artherosclerosis (Fain, 1998). Laboratory investigations of the blood glucose level as well as level of sugar or ketones in urine will help in the management of the patient's condition.

In addition, meaningful management of diabetes focuses on:
1. Diet alone and exercise, or
2. Diet with oral hypoglycaemic drugs and exercise, or
3. Diet with insulin and exercise. Exercise should however be carefully evaluated to see if the patient can tolerate it before it is recommended. Recommended daily diet regimen should be carbohydrate (60 percent), protein (15 percent), and fat (25 percent) preferably from plants and low in animal fat with an increased amount of fibre from vegetables, fruits and cereals (Standard Treatment Guidelines for Ghana, 2010).

4. Oral hypoglycaemic medication or drugs
    There are various classes of oral medication for the treatment of the condition. Oral preparations are for Type 2 patients. These are: Biguanides, Sulphonylureas and Thiazolidinediones Therapy (Standard Treatment Guidelines for Ghana, Ministry of Health, 2010).

a. **Biguanides:** An example is Metformin Hydrochloride given as 500mg-1g every 12 hours (Standard Treatment Guidelines for Ghana, Ministry of Health, 2010).

b. **Sulphonylureas:** Examples are Tolbutamide, Gliclazide, Glibenclamide and Glimepiride (Standard Treatment Guidelines for Ghana, Ministry of Health, 2010).

   i. Tolbutamide, is prescribed between "250mg-1g, every 8 to 12 hourly" (Standard Treatment Guidelines for Ghana, Ministry of Health, 2010, p. 214).

   ii. Gliclazide, in a recommended dosage between "40-160 mg every 12 hourly" (Standard Treatment Guidelines for Ghana, Ministry of Health, 2010, p. 213).

   iii Glibenclamide, which is administered on daily basis between 2.5-10mg preferably in the mornings but not exceeding 15mg daily.

   iv. Glimepiride is also given on daily basis as "2-6mg in the morning" (Treatment Guidelines for Ghana, Ministry of Health, 2010, p. 213).

c. **Thiazolidinediones Oral Therapy:** Examples are:

   i. "Pioglitazone, oral, 15-45mg, as single daily dose" (Standard Treatment Guidelines for Ghana, Ministry of Health, 2010, p. 214).

   ii. "Rosiglitazone, oral, 4-8mg, as single daily dose" (Standard Treatment Guidelines for Ghana, Ministry of Health, 2010, p. 214).

In addition to Thiazolidinediones, Metformin or a Sulphonylurea may be ordered for the patient (Standard Treatment Guidelines for Ghana, Ministry of Health, 2010).

5. Insulin Injections: In Type 1 diabetes mellitus, insulin injections are required for the rest of life of the patients (Misso et al., 2010) and are also indicated for Type 2 patients who do not respond well to oral anti-diabetic agents, pregnant diabetics as well as breast-feeding mothers whether Type 1 or 2. Insulin injection is also indicated for patients with type 2 diabetes who have severe stress such as infection, myocardial

problems as well as other recurrent conditions (Misso et al., 2010, Standard Treatment Guidelines for Ghana, Ministry of Health, 2010). Insulin injections are classified as Rapid acting, Short acting, Intermediate acting or Long acting and Pre-mixed insulin (Standard Treatment Guidelines for Ghana, Ministry of Health, 2010). Conventional Insulin Injection (CII) therapies are given as twice a day or thrice a day or as a multi-dose regimen based on the patient's condition as prescribed the physician (Razavi & Ahmadi, 2011). A much more advanced form of insulin administration is through an insulin pump, by means of which insulin is administered to a patient on regular basis depending on patient's requirements (Jeitler et al., 2008).

6. Monitoring of the Condition: Monitoring is based on self monitoring/Bedside monitoring of blood using glucometers on a daily basis or as required based on the patient's response to recommended treatment. That is, the patient can make use of a diary to record date, time and monitoring results. The diary notations may include medications, food intake, activity levels, and illness so that the patient can begin to see the relationship between blood glucose or urine ketones and treatment regimen (Fain, 1998). As patients gain flexibility and self-determination, they may manipulate insulin, diet, and exercise independently on the basis of monitoring results.

As part of the management protocol on monitoring of the blood glucose, Glycated Haemoglobin can be done on a three-month or six-month basis based on the patient's doctor's request. Glycated Haemoglobin (HBA1c) is done to find out the extent to which the patient has controlled his or her sugar intake for the past three to six months or within a particular period specified by the patient's doctor (Sikaris, 2009). Good control of diabetes is the best way to prevent or delay complications of the disease, complications that include heart disease, blindness, nerve damage and kidney damage (America Diabetes Association, 2004). The glycosylated hemoglobin test, or Hemoglobin A1c (HbA1c), is a test used to give the patient and the doctor the most accurate picture of overall diabetes control. The HbA1c test measures the amount of sugar that is attached to the haemoglobin in red blood cells, with results given as a percentage (Sikaris, 2009). Other tests can be requested as well such as fat profile and total serum protein.

7. Exercise

Exercise may be used to control blood glucose levels in individuals with Type 2 DM but when the response to these measures is inadequate, oral agents are tried. Regular, simple exercise is helpful in ensuring good glucose control. All advice on exercise must give consideration to the patient's age and the presence of complications and other medical conditions. If the patient's condition will not allow him or her to do the exercise, they should be exempted from the exercise programme (Fain, 1998).

Exercise has been found to:

1. Improve insulin sensitivity,
2. Lower blood glucose,
3. Assist with weight loss,
4. Preserve cardiovascular fitness, and
5. Improve sense of wellbeing.

8. Education: The teaching of the patient centres on the meal plan to control weight, glucose, and the lipids composition of the diet, as well as how to read nutrition labels. Performing tests accurately, interpreting test results and the monitoring and use of those results are a crucial part of patient education as well as behavioural change strategies and risk factor reduction. The benefits of exercise, preparing for exercise and the complications of exercise (such as hypoglycemia) are stressed in patient education. So by its nature, diabetes can be significantly influenced by each of these management components mentioned above (Fain, 1998). Other areas of patient teaching in diabetic care include:

1. Myths about the disease which must be dispelled through education.
2. Health history — awareness of psychosocial/emotional status, perception of the meaning of the diagnosis, how it affects the patient's life and future plans, day-to-day activities, coping mechanisms employed by the person.

Use of health care systems and community resources: planned follow ups, emergency care: patient tag, planning for travel, patient's responsibility: name and telephone numbers of her/his nurse etc. Other important aspects of care are promoting adequate nutrition, managing medication and decreasing fears of the patient regarding the unknown outcome of the condition (Reinehr and Wabittsch, 2005).

In summary, the overall treatment protocol for diabetes mellitus centres on medication, diet, exercise, monitoring and patient education which encompasses all the aspects we have already mentioned.

Major Roles of Nurses in Diabetes Care

Nurses play pivotal roles in diabetes management in hospitals. It is therefore very important for nurses to be familiar with the trends in the management of diabetes mellitus. As already pointed out in the introduction, as part of the current trend in the management of the condition, the totality of patient is paramount. This means going beyond the identification of clinical manifestations and commencement of the medical regimen by nurses. Nurses play the following specific roles in the management of patients with diabetes.

1. Screening, early diagnosis and referral of patients with diabetes mellitus.
2. Health education and dietary advice for these patients.
3. Emergency care of diabetic patients.
4. Helping in the formation of support groups for these patients.
5. Team approach.
6. Research.
7. Identifying the patient's perceived beliefs about the cause of the diabetes mellitus.

8. Identifying social meanings the patient attaches to the condition.
9. Finding out patient's reaction to the diagnosis of diabetes mellitus.
10. Finding out the patient's coping strategies for dealing with the challenges associated with the condition.

Screening, early diagnosis and referral of patients with diabetes mellitus

Nurses are among the first group of health professionals to ask their patients to be tested for diabetes mellitus. The nurse may be the first healthcare professional to suspect a patient has diabetes mellitus, prepare the patient for initial tests to be done and subsequently ask the patient to see the physician.

Health education and dietary advice for these patients

Nurses are known to have the most contact (up to 24 hours) with DM patients. This makes them well placed to educate their patients on all aspects of their diabetic care, including their health, nutrition and exercise. (Fain, 1998).

Emergency care of diabetic patients

The front-line health professionals who initiate care for patients in urgent and emergency cases are nurses. Undiagnosed or uncontrolled DM patients receive emergency care until their health status is properly evaluated and this is done by nurses. Nurses must be prepared to manage diabetic emergencies should these occur among their patients.

Team approach

The management of diabetes and its complications involves many specialists such as endocrinologists, nephrologists, neurologists, ophthalmologists, orthopaedic surgeons, paediatricians and nutritionists. (Expert Committee, 1997). In most cases during the management of patients, it is the nurse who coordinates patient care.

It is the nurse who makes sure that the patient is properly prepared to receive care from each of these specialists.

Helping in the formation of support groups for these patients

Diabetes mellitus (DM) is a chronic illness without any age limit. Support groups are particularly important for all categories of patients, especially children and older people with diabetes. A nurse can play an important and unique role in identifying support groups for patients suffering from DM. This is likely to improve their compliance with treatment and their quality of life will subsequently be affected positively.

Identifying the patient's perceived beliefs about the cause of the diabetes mellitus

Identification of patient's perceived beliefs about the cause of the DM is very imperative in the care of the patient. This will help the nurse decide on the appropriate line of intervention needed to address the patient's problem, for instance if the patient has inappropriate beliefs about the causes of the condition. The nurse will then give appropriate education to the patient to make sure that these inappropriate beliefs held by the patient are dispelled, with the overall effect of better patient compliance with the treatment (Nguma, 2010). Korsah (2011) noted that their professional training enabled nurses to give quality care to the patient in part by being able to identify and separate the patient's care needs from their lay beliefs.

Identifying social meanings the patient attaches to the condition

Social meanings that patients attach to conditions they have inform the nurse to identify appropriate forms of education for them. Social meanings attached to disease conditions are socially constructed (Kleinmann, 1988). Some meanings associated with disease conditions are socially damaging and therefore may lead to stigmatization. For instance, Abdoli (2011) identified social meanings attached to diabetes mellitus such as "defect point", "dreadful disease", "silent killer" and "worse than cancer". These meanings inform the nurse about what the patient perceives about the condition and therefore the appropriate education and information to give to the patient. Negative meanings attached to disease conditions have a negative impact on the psychological well-being of affected individuals (Schiffrin, 2001).

Finding out Patient's Reaction to the Diagnosis of Diabetes Mellitus

The patient's type of reaction to diagnosis determines the type of coping they use (Lazarus & Folkman, 1984). Similarly, the patient's reaction to diagnosis of diabetes mellitus and experiences living with it determine the type of coping strategies utilized by the patient. If nurses are able to identify the patient's reaction to diagnosis of their diabetes, it will signal the type of attention which must be given to the patient. Some of the reactions to diagnosis are inappropriate while others are appropriate. In the same vein, some of the coping strategies utilized by the patient are appropriate while some are negative. Accurate identification of these dimensions of coping used by the by patient will help the nurse in her care.

Patients' Experiences Living with Diabetes

As part of the current management protocol for diabetes mellitus, it is important for nurses to look at the living experiences of their patients and offer appropriate, comprehensive, and meaningful care to their clients. Illness brings with it a multitude of experiences, which are invariably unique to the sufferer and consequently understood in a personal way based on perspective on disease, cultural beliefs about health and illness, previous life experience including social relationships, and educational and socio-economic status. Experiences have inter-relationships between the physical and psychological body (Helman, 2000). It has also been noted that upon diagnosis of a chronic condition like diabetes, patients are confronted with a lot of challenges in all spheres of their life. The interruptions associated with illness may be centred on these specific areas: (1) Interruptions Associated with Body Self: Interruptions to 'body self' involves issues associated with sexual dysfunction and fear of complications and even death following a diagnosis of diabetes mellitus. The death of someone known to have diabetes may cause other patients to panic, and make them anxious about their condition, with thoughts of who might be next to die. This is part of the psychological trauma of living with diabetes. All these are pertinent issues which need to be addressed by the nurse.

(2) Interruptions Associated with Identity in Society: This may revolve around the negative impact of weight loss on social identity and the attribution of witchcraft to sufferers. Charmaz (1983) noted that chronic disease focuses on uncertainty in its development, progression and treatment and also forces people who are affected with the condition to relate to time in new ways. Diabetic patients experience rapid weight loss due mainly to excessive urine excretion pre-diagnosis. Some sufferers may continue to live with marked weight loss post-diagnosis due to poor diet and drug management. These patients are noted to have rapid weight loss, which is commonly associated with AIDS, a highly stigmatized condition.

(3) Interruptions Associated with Financial Circumstances:
Interruption to economic status of the patient may focus on loss of earnings, meagre salary from employers which may not be adequate for care, financial burden on families, and increased expenditure due to high cost of pharmaceutical drugs for the treatment of the condition. It is these interruptions associated with the onset of a chronic condition like diabetes that Bury (1991) termed "biographical disruptions". These constitute a significant turning point in understanding patients' experiences with chronic diseases in general.

(4) Interruptions Associated with Dietary Status: The effects of dietary change on the respondents centre on diet planning, adjustment, afford-ability, and nutritional quality of recommended foods. The difficulty of giving up preferred foods is compounded by an inability to secure the recommended food.

(5) Interruptions Associated with Normal Physiological Processes: Patients' experiences of living with diabetes may also reveal how the condition disrupts normal physiology. This can involve excessive urination and thirst, bodily weakness, vision problems and weight loss. Patients may initially perceive some of the signs and symptoms

to be normal, for example drinking too much water and urinating frequently, while later these symptoms may be viewed as abnormal and subsequently reported to the hospital for medical attention. Michael (1996) mentions that individuals with chronic diseases are confronted with losses, which implies that such patients are not able to function as before. In addition, the persons diagnosed with DM experience fluctuating feelings (Michael, 1996). Other challenges which respondents may face in living with diabetes ranges from interruption to education and work, pain of injections and boredom of taking daily oral medications, lack of equipment for glucose monitoring, and experience of particularly challenging days.

Helping Diabetics to Deal with their Living Experiences

One of the most influential works on coping with a disease condition is Lazarus and Folkman's (1984) Transactional Model of Stress Management, also known as Interactional Model of Stress Management. This suggests in that stress can be thought of as resulting from an "imbalance between demands and resources" (Lazarus & Folkman, 1984, p. 4) or as occurring when "pressure exceeds one's perceived ability to cope" (p. 4).

The model proposes two forms of appraisal, the primary and the secondary. A primary appraisal is made when the individual makes a conscious evaluation of the matter at hand of whether it is `harm` or a `loss`, a `threat` or a `challenge`. The secondary appraisal takes into consideration what the person can do to deal with challenge by evaluating the available resources. These resources may include, physical resources, such as how healthy one is, or how much energy one has, social resources, such as the family or friends one has to depend on for support in his/her immediate surroundings, psychological resources, such as self-esteem and self-efficacy, and also material resources such as how much money one has or what kind of equipment one might be able to use. Lazarus and Folkman (1984) described several methods of coping under problem-focused and emotional-focused coping strategies. Examples of problem-focused coping strategies are planning: analysing the situation to arrive at solutions to correct the problem, confrontive: assertive action taken, and seeking social support: getting practical support from friends.

In a real life situation, diabetics may utilize the primary appraisal of the cognitive component of the model to evaluate the problem at hand of whether it is harm, threat or a challenge. Then, the use of secondary appraisal by the diabetic patient focused on evaluating the coping resources around him/her. The coping resources identified by newly-diagnosed patients with diabetes may help them deal with the challenges they face including physical resources such as availability of financial resources; social resources such as the family or friends or counselors one has to depend on for support in his/her immediate surroundings; and psychological resources such as emotional support from the family and significant others. Other sources of support may be spiritual and religious support from church groups and reliance on God, drawing on medical staff for support, informational support about how to care for themselves, drawing on a diabetes patients' association for support and utilization of identity and self-empowerment among other support systems.

Other resources may include drawing on physical activity to cope with diabetes, use of humour to deal with worrisome situations, and use of surrogates for representation at meetings due to ill health. As noted already, these positive coping methods used by patients in dealing with their problems are likely to affect their quality of life. Emotion-focused coping strategies are likely to lead to poor health outcomes in individuals diagnosed with diabetes. These strategies include distancing: detaching from the situation; escape-avoidance: thinking wishfully about the situation; blaming self for the condition, having confrontations with family members and blaming them for the disease; condition, taking to alcohol and having suicidal thoughts. It is the nurse who is at the fore-front of patient care, so should be able to identify all the support systems which are available for the patient. These are extensive roles for the nurse but the current trend in the management of patients with chronic conditions including diabetes mellitus encompass all these issues discussed above. If nurses are able to employ these during patient care and management, it will go a long way to improve the quality of life of patients with diabetes.

Conclusion

In order for nurses to provide comprehensive, competent and meaningful care to patients with diabetes mellitus, nurses must understand the disease, its impact on affected individuals, and its treatment protocol. Equally important, for nurses to give comprehensive care to diabetic patients, they need to understand patients' perceptions of the socio-religio-cultural aspects of living with diabetes mellitus and their reactions to being diagnosed with the disease. Nurses should also be able to explore the living experiences of these patients in order to identify the best type of care to give them. In addition, nurses need to do primary assessment of these patients to find out what their problems are and to identify available resources to manage the problems through the secondary appraisal model of Lazarus and Folkman (1984). Quality and safe management of the patient with DM requires effective communication among different healthcare providers, including nurses of all categories.

Becoming familiar with diabetics' coping methods (positive or negative) in dealing with their problems will help nurses and other paramedical staff to empower these patients to deal successfully with diabetes in the world today.

References

Abdoli, S., Ashktorbi, T., Ahmadi, F., & Parvizy S. (2011). Diabetes Diagnosis; Disrupter Identity? *Iranian Journal of Endocrinology and Metabolism,* Vol. 13, No. 1.

American Diabetes Association (2004). Diagnosis and Classification of Diabetes Mellitus. *Diabetes Care,* 2004 (27): no. Suppl 1, s5-s10.

Bury, M. (1991). The sociology of chronic illness: a review of research and prospects. *Sociology of Health and Illness,* 13, 451-468.

Beare, P. G., & Myers, J. L. (1998). *Adult Health Nursing.* 3rd ed. New York: Mosby.

Charmaz, K. (1983). Loss of self: A fundamental form of suffering in the chronically ill. *Sociology of Health and Illness,* 5, 168-195.

Expert Committee on the Diagnosis and Classification of Diabetes Mellitus. (2003). Report of the Expert Committee on the diagnosis and classification of diabetes mellitus. *Diabetes Care,* 26, Suppl 1, S5-20.

Fain, J. A. (1998). Nursing management of adults with diabetes mellitus. In: Bear, P.G. and Myers, J. L. eds. Adult Health Nursing. 3rd ed. St. Louis: Mosby. Pp. 1406-1448.

Helman, C. G. (2000). Culture, Health, and Illness. 4th ed. Oxford: Butterworth-Heinemann.

International Diabetes Federation. (2009). *The IDF Diabetes Atlas.* 4th ed. Brussels: International Diabetes Federation 2009.

Jonanovic, L. & Pettitt, D. J. (2001). Gestational Diabetes Mellitus. *The Journal of the American Medical Association,* 286 (20): 2516-2518.

Jeitler, K., Horvath, K., Berghold, A., Gratzer, T. W., Neeser, K., Pieber, T. R., & Siebenhofer, A. (2008). Continuous Subcutaneous Insulin Infusion versus Multiple Daily Insulin Injections in Patients with Diabetes Mellitus: Systematic Review and Meta Analysis. *Diabetologia,* 51 (6): 941-51.

Kinmonth, A. & Woodcock A. (2001). Patient concerns in their first year with Type 2 diabetes: Patient and practice nurse views. *Patient Education and Counseling,* Volume 42, Number 3, March , pp. 257-270(14).

Kleinmann, A. (1988). *The Illness Narratives: Suffering, Healing, and the Human Condition.* Wilmington: Basic Books: ISBN: 0465032028.

Korsah, K. A. (2011). Nurses' stories about their interaction with clients at the Holy Family Hospital. *Open Journal of Nursing.* 1-9.

Lazarus, R. S., & Folkman, S. (1984). *Stress, Appraisal, and Coping.* New York: Springer.

Mbanya, J., Motala, A., Sobngwi, E., Assah, F., & Enoru, S. (2010). Diabetes in sub-Saharan Africa. *Lancet,* 375: 2254-2266.

Michael, S. R. (1996). Integrating chronic illness into one' life – a phenomenological inquiry. *Journal of Hoslistic Nursing,* 3, 251-267.

Misso, M. L., Egberts, K. J., Page, M., O'Connor, D., & Shaw, J. (2010). Continuous Subcutaneous Insulin Infusion (CSII) versus Multiple Insulin Injections (MI) for Type 1 Diabetes Mellitus. *Cochrane Database of Systemic Review,* 2010, 1: CD 005103.

National Diabetes Data Group. (1995). *Diabetes in America.* National Institute of Health, National Institute of Diabetes and Digestive and Kidney Diseases, NIH publication no. 95-1468, 2nd ed. Bethesda.

Nguma, L. (2010). Health-seeking and health-related behaviour for Type 2 diabetes mellitus among adults in an urban community in Tanzania.

Published PhD Thesis submitted to the University of Otago, Wellington, New Zealand.

Olshansky, S. G., Passera, D. J., & Hershow, R. C. (2005). A potential decline in life expectancy in the United States in the 21st Century. *N Engl Journal of Medicine*, 352: 1138-1145.

Reinehr, T., & Wabittsch, M. (2005). Type 2 diabetes mellitus in children and adolescents. In: Ganz, M, ed. Prevention of Type 2 Diabetes. West Sussex: John Wiley & Sons; 21-40.

Schiffrin, A. (2001). Psychosocial issues in paediatric diabetes. *Current Diabetes Report*, 1(1), 33-40.

Sikaris, K. (2009). The Correlation of Haemoglobin A1c to Blood Glucose. *Journal of Diabetes Science and Technology*, 3 (3): 429-438.

Standard Treatment Guidelines for Ghana, Ministry of Health, Ghana National Drugs Programme (GNDP), 2010.

Woodcock, A., & Kinmonth, A. L. (2001). Patient concerns in their first year with Type 2 diabetes: Patient and practice nurse views. *Patient Education and Counselling*, 42 (3), 257-270.

Razavi, Z. & Ahmadi, M. (2011). Efficacy of Thrice daily versus Twice daily Insulin Regimens on Glycohaemoglobin (HbA1c) in Type 1 Diabetes Mellitus: A Randomised Controlled Trial. *Oman Medical Journal*, 26 (1): 10-13.

Zimmet, P. (2000). Globalization, coca-colonization and the chronic disease epidemic: can the Doomsday scenario be averted? *Journal of Internal Medicine*, 247(3): 301–310.

Chapter Eleven
Trends in Stroke: Roles of Nurses and Family Caregivers
Cecilia Eliason and Patricia Avadu

Introduction

Stroke is defined simply as 'the sudden death of brain cells in a localised area due to inadequate blood flow' (on-line medical dictionary). This definition is modified by the World Health Organization (WHO) to include characteristics of Thus, a stroke or cerebrovascular accident entails "rapidly developing clinical signs of focal (at times global) disturbance of cerebral function, lasting more than 24 hours or leading to death with no apparent cause other than that of vascular origin" (WHO,1988). This definition includes signs and symptoms suggestive of ischemic and haemorrhagic strokes (intracerebral or subarachnoid).

Stroke as a Public Health Problem

Stroke is a major public health problem worldwide. It is a major cause of death second only to ischemic heart diseases (Cameron & Gignac, 2008; Larson, Franzen-Dahlin, Billing, von Arbin & Murray, 2008) and the leading cause of adult disability (Nwoso, 2001; Ogunrin, 2007). It is projected that by 2020 there will be 25 million deaths annually from cardiovascular disease worldwide, with up to19 million deaths occurring in developing countries (Lemogoun, Degante & Bovet, 2005). The incidence rate for all strokes and for stroke subtypes varies widely between and within populations. In industrialised countries of Europe and North America where half of strokes occur before age 75 years, 5,000 to 85,000 new cases of ischemic strokes occur yearly (Marsh & Keyrouz, 2010).

Currently, stroke accounts for 80 percent of deaths in adults in low-income and middle-income regions of the world (Lopez, Mathers Ezzati, Jamison & Murray, 2006; Mathers, Lopez & Murray, 2006). However, the burden of stroke and other vascular diseases is likely to increase substantially over the next few decades in these lower-income countries because of their expected health and demographic transition (Connor, Walker, Modi & Warlow, 2007). Studies conducted in South Africa, Togo and Tanzania suggest the prevalence of stroke to be between 200 and 300 per 100,000 (Connor et al., 2007; Ogunrin, 2007). In Nigeria it has been identified as the leading cause of neurological admissions in most tertiary hospitals (Nwosu, 2001).

In Ghana, cardiovascular diseases, notably hypertension and cardio-vascular accident (stroke) have become major causes of morbidity and mortality (Wiredu & Nyame, 2001). Stroke is the second biggest killer in Accra and the fifth in Ghana as whole (Morris, 2011; 'Portmouth Hospitals medics', 2012). A study by Nyame et al. (1994) showed that the proportion of death due to stroke has not changed and the mortality report from Korle Bu Teaching Hospital, Accra showed that stroke made up eleven per cent (11 percent) of autopsies from 1994 to 1998 (Wiredu & Nyame, 2001). Sixty-nine percent of stroke · patients died in less than 24 hours after onset of stroke, with higher mortality in males than in females in all age groups (Wiredu & Nyame, 2001). Agyemang et al. (2012) reported that in the Ashanti Region, the majority of stroke deaths occurred within the first seven days of admission.

A study in the 10 regions of Ghana, revealed that stroke was the fourth leading cause of death among in-patient of 32 hospitals (de-Graft Aikins, 2007) and the top cause of death at the Komfo Anokye Teaching Hospital between 2006 and 2007 (Agyeman et al., 2012). High blood pressure was found to be the most consistent and powerful predictor of stroke and is causally involved in nearly 70 percent of all stroke cases (Agyemang et al., 2012). The increasing prevalence of hypertension in Ghana, particularly in urban centres, clearly suggests that the burden of stroke will continue to increase unless urgent action is taken to halt the rising prevalence of hypertension (Agyemang, 2012; Cappucio, 2004).

Types of Stroke
There are two major types of stroke namely: ischaemic (which may be thrombotic or embolic) making up for 85 percent and haemorrhagic

(which may be intracerebral or subarachnoid) constituting 15 percent of all stroke (Albers, Amarenco, Easton et al., 2004).

A. Ischemic stroke: is a sudden loss of function resulting from disruption of the blood supply to a part of the brain, also termed as 'brain attack'. About 80 percent of all acute strokes are caused by cerebral ischemia, usually resulting from thrombotic or embolic occlusion of a cerebral artery. Ischemic strokes are subdivided into five different types based on the cause (Albers et al., 2004; Smelter, Bare, Hinkle & Cheever, 2007, pp. 2207)

Table 7.1:   Types of Ischemic Strokes

Types of stroke	Causes	Percentage
Large artery thrombotic strokes	Atherosclerotic plaques in the large blood vessels of the brain result in ischemia and infarction (deprivation of blood) to that part of the brain	20% of all strokes
Small penetrating artery thrombotic strokes (lacunar strokes)	Affects one or more vessels in the brain (microatheromatosis)	25%
Cardiogenic embolic strokes	Associated with cardiac dysrhythmias, valvular heart disease and thrombi in the left ventricle	15%
Cryptogenic strokes	Have no known cause	5 to 10 %
Strokes from other causes	Such as illicit drug use	20 to 25%

Source: Smeltzer and Brunner, 2007, pg 1888

Haemorrhagic stroke is due to occlusion of a ruptured blood vessel (haemorrhagic) or bleeding into the brain tissue, the ventricles, or the subarachnoid space. There are two subtypes:

- Primary intracerebral haemorrhage results from a spontaneous rupture of small vessels accounting for approximately 80 percent of hemorrhagic stroke and is caused by uncontrolled hypertension (Bader & Littlejohns, 2004; Smelter, Bare, Hinkle & Cheever, 2010).
- Secondary intracerebral haemorrhage is associated with arterio-venous malformations, intracranial aneurysm, intracranial neoplasm and certain medications such as anticoagulant and amphetamines (Bader & Littlejohns, 2004; Hickey 2003).

In Ghana, the proportion of death due to stroke has not changed. However, the incidence of the types of stroke is changing, with the proportion of cerebral haemorrhage which previously was on the rise declining, and that of infarction is increasing (Wiredu & Nyame, 2001).

Wiredu and Nyame (2001) in their study on stroke-related mortality at the Korle Bu teaching hospital found out that hypertension was the dominant factor of haemorrhagic stroke and an important factor in infarction while cerebral atherosclerosis was the major factor in infarction stroke.

Assessing stroke subtype in Ghana is still a challenge due to inadequate neuroimaging which is used to identify the cause of the stroke (Mensah, 2008) and as a result, only those admitted to the two teaching hospitals in Accra and Kumasi (Amosun, Nyante, & Wiredu, 2013) and the 37 Military Hospital in Accra are able to access the diagnostic investigations.

Risk Factors for Stroke

The risk of stroke doubles every 10 years after the age of 55 years, although stroke can occur in people of all ages, it is common in people over 65 years (Green & King, 2007). The factors can be divided into those that are modifiable and those that are non-modifiable. The modifiable risk factors include cardiovascular disorders, diabetes mellitus, sickle cell disease, hyperlipidemia (high blood cholesterol), unhealthy lifestyle behaviours such as smoking, increased alcohol consumption, drug abuse, sedentary lifestyle, obesity and geographical location and socioeconomic conditions (World Health Organization, 2002).

Findings of the INTERSTROKE study (a study of risk factors for stroke in low- and middle-income countries) showed that five risk factors accounted for more than 80 percent of the global risk of all stroke (ischaemic and intracerebral haemorrhagic). These are hypertension, current smoking, abdominal obesity, diet, and lack of physical activity (O'Donnel et al., 2010). For ischemic stroke, the study recorded a significant association among the five mentioned risk factors in addition to five other identified risk factors namely, lack of physical activity, diabetes mellitus, alcohol intake, psychosocial factors, and apolipoproteins (O'Donnell et al., 2010).

Another cardiovascular disorder, atrial fibrillation (AF), is also a risk factor for stroke. Hart et al., (2004) found that AF is a strong, independent risk factor for ischemic stroke. Most strokes in patients with AF are cardio-embolic, caused by an embolism of the left atrial appendage.

Diabetes is another risk factor. According to the Framingham Study (Kanel & McGee, 1979), persons with diabetes have double the risk of stroke as persons without diabetes. Persons with Type 1 diabetes have an increased incidence of atherogenic risk factors such as hypertension, obesity, and abnormal blood lipid panels (Goldstein et al., 2001). Current estimates indicate that about 150 million people have Type 2 diabetes globally and are also at risk of developing stroke. Although diabetes is treatable, the presence of the disease increases a person's chance of developing stroke (Reddy & Yusuf, 1998; Zumo, 2007).

Sickle cell disease involves the clamping of blood cells and subsequent blockage of blood vessels, thereby increasing the chance of developing stroke (American Heart Association, 2007). In sickle cell disease, the increased haemolysis and altered rheological properties of RBCs are responsible for development of ischemic stroke (Lemogoum, Degaute & Bovet, 2005) in most young adults under 20 who are suffering from sickle cell anaemia.

The American Heart Association (2007) reported that people with high blood cholesterol are at a higher risk of having stroke therefore effective control of hyperlipidemia reduces this risk.

Regarding socioeconomic, factors both men and women who fall within the low socioeconomic groups are exposed to greater social and health disadvantage (Avendano et al., 2006). Studies show that stroke is more common among people within the low socioeconomic group (AHA, 2007).

Apart from economical factors' low educational level also has been associated with increase stroke incidence among people aged 65 to 74 years. However, in people aged above 75 years, higher socioeconomic factors have been linked with a higher incidence of stroke (Avendano et al., 2006).

Unhealthy lifestyle factors include excessive alcohol consumption, drug abuse, cigarette smoking and physical inactivity. Excessive consumption of alcohol increases the incidence of stroke. On the other hand, reduced consumption of alcohol is associated with reduced risk of developing coronary heart disease.

Cigarette smoking, according to Lemogoum, Degaute and Bovet (2005), doubles the risk of developing stroke. Studies have shown that while tobacco use in developed countries is on the decrease, the opposite is observed in developing countries (Lemogoum, Degaute & Bovet, 2005). This is not surprising as the developing countries have become the major target of transnational tobacco industries and they have weak or non-existence tobacco control programmes. Drug addiction is a chronic relapsing disorder associated with some societal health related problems. Among the drugs that are misused are heroin, cocaine and amphetamines and these have been associated with risk of developing stroke. It is also documented that oral contraceptive use combined with cigarette smoking also increases the stroke risk (AHA, 2007).

Non-modifiable risk factors include, gender, genetic traits, ethnicity and age. Morbidity of stroke increases with age and as a result, the chances of a person developing stroke doubles for each decade of life after 55 years (AHA, 2007; Howard et al., 1995; Zumo, 2006) had reported that 95 percent of strokes are found in people age 45 years and older. Increasing age has been reported to be the strongest risk factor for cerebral infarction, primary intra-cerebral and sub-arachnoid bleeding (Gavras, 2005). This does not imply that stroke cannot occur in people below those ages for stroke can occur in any age, including foetuses (Brain Basics, 2010).

In sub-Saharan Africa, most cases of stroke occur in relatively young people (mean age < 60 years in most studies), some 10-15 years younger than stroke patients in developed countries (Bonita & Truelsen, 2003). The age of occurrence is even younger for hemorrhagic stroke than for ischaemic stroke. The peak age of fatal haemorrhagic stroke was 50-59 years and that of ischemic was 60-69 years (Walker and McLarry, 1995).

Men are 1.25 percent more likely to suffer from stroke than women although women comprise 60 percent of deaths from stroke (Thorogood et al. 2007). Attah-Agyepong, (2008) also reported that the overall male-to-female ratio is 2:1. This confirms that the incidence of stroke is higher in men even though more women die from it than men (Ogurin, 2008). This may be because on the average, women are older when they develop stroke. The risk factors for women include pregnancy, childbirth, hormonal replacement, menopause and the use of certain contraceptives (AHA, 2007).

The risk of death from stroke is found to be higher in African Americans than in white Americans. The risk of developing stroke is higher if a parent, grandparent, sister or brother has had it (Gillum, 1999; AHA, 2007).

The major risk factors for stroke directly influence incidence and indirectly affect case fatality. Therefore, the identification and understanding of the magnitude of these stroke determinants will go a long way in stroke management (Ogurin, 2007).

Pathophysiology of Stroke

With ischaemic stroke, the cerebral arteries become blocked as result of embolus or thrombus, auto-regulatory mechanisms help maintain cerebral circulation until collateral circulation develops to deliver blood to the affected area. Obstruction of blood flow to the brain lasting for more than four minutes causes oxygen deprivation, which leads to infarction of brain tissue. Neurons served by the occluded vessel die from lack of oxygen and nutrients, resulting in cerebral infarction.

Accumulation of calcium, sodium and water in the injured cells leads to release of excitatory neurotransmitters causing further cell injury and swelling. The size of the area of inadequate perfusion in the brain results in disruption of motor, sensory, cranial nerve and cognitive functions.

When haemorrhage is the cause, impaired cerebral perfusion causes infarction and the blood itself acts as a space-occupying lesion mass. The brain's regulatory mechanism attempts to maintain equilibrium by increasing blood pressure. This is to maintain cerebral perfusion pressure. The increased intracranial pressure (ICP) forces cerebrovascular fluid (CSF) out, thereby impairing absorption and circulation, leading to damaged brain cells.

Clinical Manifestations

A stroke may involve signs and symptoms such as weakness, numbness, headache, speech abnormalities (including both aphasia and dysarthria), mental status change, vision changes, falling or trouble walking, and dizziness or vertigo (Kleindofer et al., 2010). However, the manifestations stated may be affected by gender. According to Barret (2007), a greater proportion of women presented with weakness than men, though no gender difference was found in numbness, visual deficits, or language. In another study, Jerath et al. (2011) using 4,499 patients found that women presented with coma, paralysis, aphasia, swallowing problems, and urinary incontinence more frequently than men. Dysphasia is another common sign which, according to Koeneker (2003), is seen more in women than men. With respect to ischaemic stroke, a key difference noticed is that women present with non-traditional symptoms such as generalized weakness, fatigue, mental status change, and disorientation (Jerath, 2011). However, survivors of major strokes were found to have been left with considerable disability. Even those with minor strokes were found to have symptoms such as mental fatigue, problems with concentration and memory irritability, emotional liability and intolerance to stress.

These are termed 'hidden or invisible disabilities' (Green & King, 2007).

A stroke may involve sudden numbness or weakness of the face, arm, or leg, especially on one side of the body that usually resolves in a few minutes. Other symptoms include difficulty speaking or understanding speech, difficulty seeing with one or both eyes, loss of balance or coordination, severe headache with no known cause and fainting or unconsciousness. Fever is usually associated with poor outcome in patients with acute ischemic stroke, and proper treatment and assessment must be done (Alberts, 2001).

Diagnostic investigations

Diagnostic investigation for stroke includes computerised tomography (CT), magnetic resonance imaging (MRI), or cerebral angiography of the brain. These are done within three weeks of the cerebral event (Smeltzer, Baer, Hinkle & Cheever, 2007; Bader & Littlejohns, 2004).

Computerised tomography (CT) imaging is the most reliable for determining type of stroke. In many hospitals, CT scan is only performed in about 50 percent of all patients presenting with stroke (Kengne and Anderson, 2006). In Ghana, currently (2013), there are four health institutions that, provide this test at a cost of GH¢500.00 per session and this is not covered by the National Health Insurance Scheme (NHIS).

Stroke Management and Treatment

Initial management of the patient with stroke is aimed at early diagnosis and early identification of the client who can benefit from thrombolytic treatment. This is also directed at preserving cerebral oxygenation, preventing complications, stroke recurrence and rehabilitating the patient.

Stroke is an emergency and requires early intervention to prevent complications and reduce mortality. Management of stroke is in three phases: the acute phase which includes transportation to the emergency unit, neuro-intensive and stroke unit management; the sub-acute phase management, which is mainly supportive and takes place in the ward and physiotherapy unit. The chronic phase takes place in the community and at outpatient clinics (Odusote, 2007).

In the acute phase, initial assessment of the client is done. This includes: collection of health history including demographic data; maintenance of patent airway to ensure oxygenation to the brain; administration of oxygen to nourish the brain cells; monitoring of vital signs such as blood pressure, pulse, respiration and temperature to identify physiological changes, with special attention to blood pressure; monitoring of level of consciousness to determine the extent of neurological problems; monitoring pupillary response to light to exclude damage to the brain stem; movement of extremities to determine level of paralysis, which involves testing of motor reflexes; and loss of sensation in the affected part of the body (LeMone & Burke, 2004).

Treatment approaches to acute ischaemic stroke include; reperfusion strategies, antiplatelet therapy, anticoagulant and combination therapy.

Reperfusion Strategy and Thrombolytic Agent: The drug of choice is recombinant tissue plasminogen activator (rt-PA) which is potent in adults for improving neurologic recovery and reducing disability. This drug increases blood viscosity thereby reducing oedema. It is administered within three hours after onset of stroke and contraindicated in more than three hours after onset of stroke. Antiplatelet therapy is useful for acute treatment and chronic prevention of ischaemic stroke. The drug of choice is Aspirin, with a dosage of 160 to 300mg/day starting 48 hours after onset of neurologic symptoms and continuing for 2 to 4 hours. Aspirin therapy results in a reduction of 9 to 10 deaths or recurrent strokes per 1,000 treated patients (Marsh & Keyrouz, 2010). Recovery from stroke is often slow and incomplete, leading to partial or complete loss of locomotion, activities of daily living (ADL), cognition and communication skills (Nair & Taly, 2002).

When the patients are out of the acute phase they need to be admitted on the ward to ensure that they are fully stabilized. On the ward, the nurse is the main cadre for ensuring the day-to-day care to full recovery and rehabilitation. The length of stay on admission varies substantially according to region and affordability. The median hospital stay in developed countries was only three days whilst there is very little information on specialised stroke-unit care in developing countries (Brainin, Teuschl, & Kalra, 2007).

Roles of the Nurse

Most stroke victims do not seek early medical attention due to lack of recognition of signs and symptoms and risk factors of stroke (Yoon & Byles, 2002). Although many people who suffer stroke recover fully, a significant number are left with disabilities that affect their physical, emotional, interpersonal and family status (Lemone & Burke, 2004). In Ghana stroke is a major burden not only on patients and family but also on medical staff and the health-care system (Gould, 2011; Morris, 2011). Nursing management of stroke involves multiple steps designed to ensure that patients receive appropriate, rapid and efficient care (Alberts, 2001). This step involves curative, rehabilitative and preventive activities.

The acute phase of stroke is often the time when most of the curative care is rendered to stabilize the patient. The nurse is responsible for the initial assessment of the stroke patient, which includes level of consciousness, patency of the airway, respiratory status, blood pressure, and heart rate. A blood glucose determination is performed to rule out hypoglycaemia or hyperglycaemia, which can mimic a stroke or potentiate ischaemic injury (White et al., 2011). In addition, nurses provide quality nursing care based on the identified needs of the stroke patients, in collaboration with other members of the health team. These includes monitoring and documentation of vital signs, provision of safety measures such as aspiration precautions, fall precautions, use of restraints, seizure precautions. Provision of comfort measures to the stroke patient includes frequent linen changes, maintenance of personal hygiene, turning and proper positioning of patient.

Nursing assessment plays a vital role in the early assessment and initiation of stroke care. Admission into dedicated stroke beds with bed accessories for positioning of the stroke patient and early swallow assessment are done to prevent aspiration are some of the interventions initiated by the nurse. It is evident that the majority of stroke patients respond to simple nursing interventions (Adams et al., 2007). Thus, the nurse provides interventions to maintain body functions and prevent complications. Nursing care is given based on patient's condition, needs and priorities. Until recently, stroke patients at the Korle Bu Teaching Hospital and Ridge Hospital in Ghana, were managed in the same medical unit as patients diagnosed with other medical conditions, without receiving special stroke care. The development of a multidisciplinary stroke unit at Korle Bu and Ridge hospitals therefore, is the first strategic effort needed to improve stroke outcome and prevent complications (Moris, 2011).

Physician specialists from Korle Bu and Ridge hospitals in their efforts to improve the outcome of stroke and prevent complications, collaborated with stroke specialists from the United Kingdom to establish multidisciplinary stroke team at Korle Bu hospital (Morris, 2011). A follow-up on this collaboration led to interprofessional discussions and workshops on the implementation of current and best practices stroke care in Ghana. At these workshops it was decided that as part of finding solutions and sustaining change, clinical development should include introduction of swallowing assessment, dietetic input, current positioning and handling of patient to improve recovery and prevent secondary complication (Gould, 2011). Presently, stroke patients admitted in the acute phase are managed by identified stroke professionals to improve their care and prevent early complication. Health professionals comprising medical, nursing, and physiotherapist have been identified in the polyclinics, emergency rooms as clinical leads for the proposed multidisciplinary stroke team. Most of these interventions are done by the nurses in collaboration with the team.

Stroke rehabilitation is the restoration of patients to their previous or near previous physical, mental, and social capability. This involves a team made up of physiotherapist, speech therapist and occupational therapist. The role of the nurse involves assisting the patient towards maximum functional capacity and involving the patient's family and significant others in the decision making and care plan. The nurse also provides guidelines for home care, involves the patient in lifestyle modification and assists the patient in accepting and adapting to disability by providing emotional support (Guidelines for nursing management of stroke..., 2013). Most often, nurses initiate rehabilitation upon admission, by assisting the patient in the performance of activities of daily living in collaboration with other health team members. In addition, in the absence of a physiotherapist and occupational therapist in the ward, nurses are expected to carry out their work. Apart from these people, nurses also assume the roles of other team members such as the speech therapist, by assisting patients to speak or communicate independently . In so doing, nurses are often seen as the coordinators of the team and a central point for communication and decision making. Hence nurses plays an important role in the rehabilitative phase. The nurse performs pre-discharge needs assessment which helps to identify the post-discharge physical, emotional, social and financial needs of the patient.

In order to continue care in the community, the nurse involves the family or close relatives in the discharge planning to help the patient integrate fully. It should be emphasized that physical function may continue to improve for up to three months and speech may continue to improve for even longer. Also, the family caregiver is given structured information on the care of the patient before discharge. Education and information on caring for the stroke patient given to the family caregiver help to prevent complications and promote adherence to long term medication and rehabilitation in the community (Brainin, Teuschl, & Kalra, 2007). To ensure safety and community access, the nurse coordinates with the community health nurse to assess the client's home.

In the prevention stage, the nurse's role involves provision of education on the condition, causes and risk factors, recognition of early signs and symptoms and lifestyle modification. Follow up is important and the family caregiver needs to take time off and seek help from respite care services to look after their own health.

Role of Family Caregivers of Stroke Patients

About 50-75 percent of stroke victims can recover to some degree and most of the recovery tends to occur during the first six months following an acute stroke (Hickey, 1997; Gresham, Duncan & Stason, 1995). The time needed for stroke care is always long and extends beyond the hospital boundary. Most stroke survivors rely on family caregivers to assist them with the physical, cognitive, behavioural and emotional changes commonly associated with a stroke (National Stroke Association-NSA, 2002).

With up to 80 percent of stroke patients returning to the community (Anderson, Linto & Stewart-Wynne, 1995), the support of family caregivers would play a key role in determining the success of rehabilitation. The consequences of a stroke as well as the rehabilitation of stroke patients have become important in the health delivery system. The increasing recognition of the role that caregivers play for stroke survivors in the community means, in practical terms, involving them in care planning and giving them training appropriate for their caring role (Cecil et al ., 2009). The first month of caring for a stroke survivor has been identified as being stressful, with problems such as safety of the stroke patient, difficulty in managing activities of daily living and coping with cognitive, behavioural and emotional disabilities of the patients (Eliason, unpublished data; Grants et al., 2004).

Initially, family caregivers often experience difficulty in coping with the unknown, and uncertainty in solving problems and making decisions about the care of stroke survivors. Although individuals manage problems every day, newness of the caregiver role combined with fear may unknowingly harm stroke survivors by their actions (Hanger & Mulley, 1993).

To improve the quality of life of the stroke patient and that of the family caregiver, early recognition of the caregiver and education on care of the patient is important. The importance of quality of life after stroke is widely acknowledged in developed countries, but this approach is still lacking in developing countries (like Ghana) because it requires a team effort involving many people as well as the patient and importantly, the family caregiver. Furthermore, family caregivers of stroke patients play an influential role in promoting successful rehabilitation of stroke survivors (Eliason, unpublished data).

Learning to live with and to take care of a family member with stroke is very complex and demanding (Sit, Wong, Clinton, Li & Fong, 2004). Caregivers experience some loss in terms of assuming unfamiliar roles and responsibilities, little or no freedom to do things without consulting or thinking of others, and changes in relationship with friends and relatives and even loss of friends (Grant & Davis,

1997). A study by Berg et al. (2005) found that 38 percent of spousal carers were exhausted at six months and 29 percent at 18 months with an increased incidence of depression among aged spousal carers. Hence the provision of education on care of stroke patients would go a long way to lessen the burden on stroke caregivers.

The stroke survivors after discharge from the hospital are also faced with environmental barriers that hinder their integration in the community. A study done in Rwanda (Urimbenshi & Rhoda, 2011) identified physical barriers for stroke patients such as inaccessible entrances and exits to buildings; social barriers such as lack of social support and attitudinal barriers included negative behaviour such as stigma which stroke survivors have to deal with in order to re-integrate in their community.

The economic impact of stroke can be felt both as cost to the country's health care system as well as the loss of income and production of those affected either directly by the disease or indirectly as caregivers to those with stroke (Agyemang et al., 2012). Maintaining the patients in the community may be ideal but it is not without cost. This cost could be associated with a range of negative experiences including emotional crisis, physical discomfort, guilty feeling, anxiety, and feeling of social isolation, depression, hopelessness, and financial difficulties (Andersen et al., 2000; Teel, Duncan, & Lai, 2001; White, Poissant, Coté-LeBlanc, & Wood-Dauphinee, 2006; Eliason, unpublished data)

Although the physical, psychological, emotional, and social consequences of care giving and its economic benefit to society are well recognized (Wade et al., 2002; Scholte et al., 1998), caregivers' needs are often given low priority in the management of stroke in Africa. It is the responsibility of the nurse to recognize the signs and intervene before the client is discharged home. Family caregivers need to be taught by health professionals how to cope with stress (time management, progressive muscle relaxation, etc). so as to reduce the negative impact of stress, depression and physical exhaustion on their health. Nurses need to create time for caregivers to help alleviate the caregiving burden on them by having a support group that meets often, when the stroke patient is brought for physiotherapy sessions. The dependence on unpaid caregivers to support individuals with disability to live in the community needs to be accompanied by a responsible strategy to support these caregivers in adapting to and managing their new roles.

Provision of information on stroke and how to manage its disabilities would go a long way to help the caregivers. Family caregivers should get involved with basic physiotherapy training to help them support the patient at home. Support groups with audiovisual materials should be made available for family caregivers. Family caregivers with experience can offer counselling intervention to potential caregivers.

Education on behavioural modification and medical therapies during hospitalisation by specialists using simple messages adapted to patients' education and cultural background may be an opportunity to increase adherence to secondary prevention measures. The family has an important role in continuity of care and should be included in health education to encourage and help patients with drug intake and lifestyle changes.

Conclusion

Stroke is a major public health problem and survival of the stroke patient will depend mainly on well-trained stroke nurses who are capable of managing the stroke patient in the acute, subacute and chronic phases. With the majority of the stroke survivors returning to the community, the role of family caregivers becomes important, especially in managing the emotional, physical and socioeconomic problems associated with stroke.

References

Adams, H.P. Jr., del Zoppo G., Alberts, M.J., Bhatt, D.L., Brass, L., Furlan, A. ... Wijdicks, F.M. (2007). Guidelines for the early management of adults with ischemic stroke: *Circulation*; 115:e478–534. doi: 10.1161.

Andersen, H.E., Schultz-Larsen, K., Kreiner, S., Forchhammer, B.H., Driksen, K. & Brown, A., (2000). Can readmission after stroke be prevented? Results of a randomized clinical study: A postdischarge follow-up service for stroke survivors. *Stroke*; 31:1038–1045.

Addo, J., Smeeth L., & Leon D.A., (2008) Prevalence, Detection, Management and Control of Hypertension in Ghanaian Civil Servants. *Eth. Dis* Autumn; 18:505-11.

Agyeman, C., Attah-Adjepong, G., Owusu-Dabo, E., De-Graft Aikins A., Addo J., Edusei K., Nkum B.C., & Ogedegbe G. (2012). Stroke in Ashanti Region of Ghana. *Ghana Medical Journal. 46.2*

Agyemang, C., & Owusu-Dabo, E. (2008). Prehypertension in the Ashanti Region of Ghana, West Africa: an opportunity for early prevention of clinical hypertension. *Public Health* 122:19-24

Agyemang, C. (2006) Rural and urban differences in blood pressure and hypertension in Ghana, West Africa. *Public Health*; 120: 522-33.

Albers, G.W., Amarenco, P., Easton, D. J. et al. (2004) Antithrombotic and thrombolytic therapy for ischaemic stroke. The seventh ACCP conference on thrombolytic therapy. *Chest 126*: 4835-5125.

Amosun, S. L., Nyante, G. G., & Wiredu, E. K. (2013). Perceived and experienced restrictions in participation and autonomy among adult survivors of stroke in Ghana. *African Health Sciences, 13*(1), 24–31. doi:10.4314/ahs.v13i1.4.

Appelros, P., Nydevik I & Terent A (2006) Living setting and utilisation of ADL assistance one year after a stroke with special reference to gender differences. *Disability & Rehabilitation 28*, 43–49.

Attah-Adjepong, G., (2008) A retrospective descriptive study on cerebrovascular accidents at the Komfo Anokye Teaching Hospital (KATH) in Kumasi. MPhil thesis unpublished.

Avendano, M., Kawachi, I., Lenthe, F.V., Boshuizen, H.C., Mackenbach, J.P., Vanden Bos G.A.M., Fay, M.E., & Berkman L. F. (2006). Socioeconomic status and stroke incidence in the US elderly: The role of risk factors in EPESE study. *Stroke*; 37:1368-73.

Barrett, K. M., Brott, T. G. & Brown, R. D. J. (2007). Ischemic Stroke Genetics Study Group: Sex differences in stroke severity, symptoms, and deficits after first ever ischemic stroke. Journal Stroke Cerebrovasc Di; 16:34-39.

Bonita R. & Truelsen T., (2003). Reflection and Reaction. Stroke in sub-Saharan Africa: a neglected chronic disease. *The Lancet Neurology* 2(10).

Bovet, P. (2002). The cardiovascular disease epidemic: global, regional, local. *Trop Med Int Health* 7: 717–21.

Brainin, M., Teuschl, Y. & Kalra, L. (2007). Acute treatment and long-term management of stroke in the developing world. *The Lancet Neurology* 6:533-561.

Cameron, J.I. & Gignac, M.A.M. (2008). 'Timing it right': A conceptual framework for addressing the support needs of family caregivers to stroke survivors from the hospital to the home. *Journal of Patient Education and Counselling* 70, 305–314.

Cappucio, F. P, Micah, F. B. et al. (2004). Prevalence, Detection Management and Control of Hypertension in Ashanti, *West Africa Hypertension 43*; 1017-22.

Cecil, R., Parahoo, K., Thompson, K., McCaughan, E., Power, M. & Campbell, Y. (2010). 'The hard work starts now': a glimpse into the lives of carers of community-dwelling stroke survivors. *Journal of Clinical Nursing 20*: 1723-1730

Connor, M.D., Walker, R., Modi, G & PWarlow C., (2007) Burden of stroke in black population in Sub-Saharan Africa. *Lancet Neurology* 6:269-75.

de-Graft Aikins, A. (2007) Ghana's neglected chronic disease epidemic: A developmental challenge. *Ghana Medical journal* 41:154-159.

Eliason, C. (2008). 'Experiences of family caregivers of stroke patients. A study at the Accra Metropolis' MPhil thesis submitted to the University of Ghana, 2008.

Goldstein, L. B., Adams, R., Becker, K., et al. (2001) Primary prevention of ischemic stroke: a statement for healthcare professionals from the Stroke Council of the American Heart Association. *Circulation:103* (1):163-182.

Gould, A., Asare, H., Akpalu, A., Cullen, L., Easton, S., Jarrett, D., Johnson, L., Kirk, H., Spice C, Williams J. (2011). Development of stroke care in Ghana. *International Journal Stroke.* (2):150-1. doi: 10.1111/j.1747-4949.2010.00571.x.

Hart, R.G., Pearce, L.A., Koudstaal, P.J. (2004). Transient ischemic attacks in patients with atrial fibrillation -- implications for secondary prevention: the European Atrial Fibrillation Trial and Stroke Prevention in Atrial Fibrillation III Trial. *Stroke*; 35 (4):948-951.

Guidelines for the NURSING MANAGEMENT OF STROKE PATIENTS accessed 16[th]May 2013 from http:www.strokesocietyphil.org/files. chapter 8.pdf.

Howard, G., Evans G.W., Pearce, K., Howard, V.J., Bell, R.A., Mayer, E.J. & Burke, G.L. (1995). Is the stroke belt disappearing? An analysis of racial, temporal, and age effects. *Stroke*; 26:1153-1158.

Howson, C.P., Reddy, K.S., Ryan, T.J., & Bale, J.R., (1998). *Control of Cardio-vascular Diseases in Developing Countries: Research, Development, and Institutional Strengthening.* Washington, DC: National Academy Press.

Lavados, P.M., Sacks, C., Prina, L. et al. (2005). Incidence, 30-day case fatality rate and prognosis of stroke in Iquique, Chile: A 2-year community based prospective study. *Lancet* 365:2206-11.

Larson, J., Franzen-Dahlin, A., Billing, E., von Arbin, M., Murray, V. & Wredling, R. (2008). The impact of gender regarding psychological well-being and general life situation among spouses of stroke patients during the first year after the patients' stroke event: a longitudinal study. *International Journal of Nursing Studies 45*, 257–265.

Lemogoum, D., Degante, J.P. & Bovet, P. (2005). Stroke prevention, treatment and rehabilitation in sub-Saharan Africa. *American Journal of Preventive Medicine. 29*; 95-101.

LeMone, P., & Burke, K. (2008). *Medical-Surgical Nursing Critical thinking in client care.* 4th ed. Upper Saddle River: Pearson Prentice Hall.

Lopez, A. D., Mathers, C. D., Ezzati, M., Jamison, D. T. and Murray, C. J. L. (2001). Global and regional burden of disease and risk factors,: systematic analysis of population health data. *Lancet* 2006; 367: 1747–57.

Marsh, J.D. & Keyrouz, S.G. (2010). Stroke prevention and treatment. *Journal of the American College of Cardiology* 56 (9)

Mayo, N.E., Wood-Dauphinee, S., Robert, C., Durcan, L. and Carlton, J. (2002). Activity, participation and quality of life 6 months post stroke. *Archives of Physical Medicine and Rehabilitation* 83, 1035-1042.

Mathers, C. D., Lopez, A. D. & Murray C. J. L. (2006). The burden of disease and mortality by condition: data, methods and results for 2001. In: Lopez, A.D., Mathers, C.D., Ezzati, M., Murray, C.J.L., Jamison, D.T. eds. *Global burden of disease and risk factors.* New York: Oxford University Press, 45–240.

Mensah, G. A. (2008). Epidemiology of stroke and high blood pressure in Africa. *Heart, 94*(6), 697–705.

Morris, K. (2011). Collaboration works to improve stroke outcomes in Ghana. *International Journal of Stroke* 377: 1681-1693. DOI:10.1111/j.1747-4949.2010.00571.x.

Nair, K. P. & Taly, A.B. (2002). Stroke rehabilitation: traditional and modern approaches. *Neurol India 50*: S85–93.

Nyame, P.K., Bonsuh Bruce, N., Amoah, A.G.B., Agyei, S., Nyarko, E., Amuah, E.A. & Biritwum, R.B.(1994). Current trends in the incidence of cardiovascular accident in Accra. *West Africa Medical Journal Journal* 13:183-186

Nwosu, C.M., Nwabueze, A.C., Ikeh, V.O. (2002). Stroke at the prime of life: a study of Nigerian Africans between the ages of 16 and 45 years. *East Afr Med J.* Jul; 69(7):384-90.

Ogurin A.O. (2007) Recent advances in the management of cerebrovascular accident. *Benin Journal of Postgraduate Medicine* 9 Vol. 9(1).

Olawale, O.A, Jaya S.I., Anigbogu, C.N., Appiah-Kubi, K.O. & Jones-Okai, (2011). Exercise training improves walking function in an African group of stroke survivors: A randomized controlled trial. *Clinical Rehabilitation* 25:442.

Portsmouth Hospitals Medics helping to improve stroke care in Ghana (2012). Available at: http://www.porthosp.nhs.uk/default.aspx. locid-094new0gd.Lang-EN.htm. [Accessed 25 February 2013].

Pusser, B. E., Robertson, S.L., Robinson, M.D., Barton, C., Dobson, L. A. (2005). Stroke prevention in atrial fibrillation: are we following the guidelines? *N C Medical Journal,* 66 (1):9-13.

Reddy, K.S., Yusuf, S. (1998). Emerging epidemic of cardiovascular disease in developing countries. *Circulation.*; 97:596- 601).

Smeltzer, S.C., Bare, B.G., Hinkle, J.L. & Cheever, K.H. (2007) *Brunner and Suddarth's Textbook of Medical-Surgical Nursing.* 11th ed. Philadelphia: Lippincott Williams & Wilkins.

Teel, C.S., Duncan, P., Lai, S.M., (2001). Caregiving experiences after stroke. *Nursing Research* ;50 (1):53–56.

The Seventh Report of the Joint National Committee on Prevention, Detection, Evaluation and Treatment of High Blood Pressure. (2003, December). NIH Publication No. 03-5233. *Hypertension,* 2003;42:1206. Available at: http://www.nhlbi.nih.gov/guidelines/hypertension/.

Thorogood, M., Connor, M., Tollman, S., Hundt, G.L., Fowkes, G., & Marsh J. (2007). Cross-sectional study of vascular risk factors in a rural South African population: Data from the South African Stroke Prevention Initiative. *Public Health*; 7:326 doi:10.1186/1471-2458-7-326.

Urimbenshi, G., & Rhoda, A. (2011). Environmental barriers experienced by stroke patients in Musanze district in Rwanda: a descriptive qualitative study. *African Health Sciences* 11:234-245.

Vorster H. H. (2002). The emergence of cardiovascular disease during urbanisation of Africans. *Public Health Nutrition*; 5: 239–43

Walker, R.W. & McLarry, D. G., (1995). Hypertension and stroke in developing countries. *Lancet* 346.

White, C.J., Abou-Chebl, A., Ctes, C.U., Levy E.L., McMullan, P.W., Rocha-Singh, K., Weinbegern, J. M., & Wholey, M.K., (2011). Stroke intervention on catheter based therapy for acute ischaemic stroke. *Journal of American College of Cardiology: 58.*

White, C.L., Poissant, L., Coté-LeBlanc, G., Wood-Dauphinee, S. (2006). Long-term caregiving after stroke: The impact on caregivers' quality of life. *Journal of Neuroscience Nursing; 38* (5):354–360.

Wiredu, E.K., & Nyame, P.K. (2001) Stroke-related mortality at Korle Bu Teaching Hospital, Accra, Ghana. *East African Medical Journal*; 78:180–4.

World Health Organization. (2002). *The World Health Report.* Geneva: WHO.

World Health Organization. (2011). WHO action plan for the strategy for prevention and control of non communicable: Cardiovascular diseases, Facts Sheet No. 317. Available at: http://www.who.int/mediacentre/factsheets/fs317/en/index.html. [Accessed 18 December 2012.]

World Health Organization. (1997). The World Health Report: conquering suffering, enriching humanity Geneva: World Health Organization.

WHO MONICA Project Investigators (1988). The World Health Organization MONICA Project (Monitoring trends and determinants in cardiovascular disease). *Journal of Clinical Epidemiol* 41, 105-114.

Zumo, A.L., (2006). What is stroke? How to recognize, prevent and treat stroke. *The Perspective.*

Chapter Twelve
Nursing Research: A Focus on Qualitative Orientation and Application

Lydia Aziato and Kwadwo Ameyaw Korsah

Introduction

Research forms the bedrock of evidence-based practice and the provision of effective nursing care draws heavily on rigorous nursing research. Thus, nursing research involves the use of systematic and verifiable processes for investigating a particular phenomenon. Research conducted by nurses has increased over the years following the introduction of higher degree programmes in nursing. At its inception, nursing research drew from other disciplines since nurses obtained higher degrees from other disciplines and they therefore applied the knowledge obtained from these disciplines in nursing research. Therefore, the knowledge derived from these research activities were seen as borrowed knowledge (Algase & Whall 1993). Indeed, nursing is considered a young profession and the use of borrowed knowledge in the discipline of nursing has created some discourse on the authenticity of nursing as a discipline with a distinct body of knowledge (Heitkemper, 2007). It cannot be over-emphasized that nurses with the requisite academic preparation need to undertake research within all domains of nursing to enhance knowledge development for the discipline of nursing.

There are two main research paradigms employed by social science investigators including nurses. These qualitative and quantitative paradigms have unique epistemological and ontological assumptions and they view the world from different perspectives. The quantitative paradigm focuses on numbers, statistical analysis, and a highly structured and controlled research process with an aim of generalizability. Data are collected in quantitative studies through questionnaires, structured interviews, observations, and other measuring tools. On the contrary, qualitative research focuses on word, meaning or understanding through the use of open-ended questions, and flexible designs aimed at understanding why and how a phenomenon exists within a particular context. In qualitative research, data may be collected through naturalistic observations, semi-structured or unstructured interviews, focus group discussions, self-reflection, and case studies and the researcher can use a range of interconnected methods during the study. Nurses may also engage in mixed methods research and base their research decisions on pragmatism (Denzin & Lincoln, 1998; Nelson, Treichler, & Grossberg, 1992; Silverman, 2001). The choice of a particular orientation depends on the type of research question(s) to be answered. For example the researcher may employ purely quantitative, qualitative, or mixed methods depending on the type of research questions to be addressed.

Philosophical Underpinnings of Nursing Research

Major meta-theoretical frameworks or paradigms that guide social research including nursing research are positivist, interpretivist and critical paradigms (Patton, 1990). The positivist paradigm has a strong link to quantitative research; and qualitative studies align with the interpretivist paradigm. In this chapter, the terms meta-theoretical framework, philosophical underpinning, and research paradigms are used interchangeably to represent paradigms or worldviews that guide social research. Although some authors try to differentiate these terminologies, they all conclude that these paradigms drive a particular research and a researcher aligns the study to a particular orientation (paradigm) based on the purpose or goal of the study (Guba & Lincoln, 1994; LeCompte & Schensul, 1999; Patton, 2002).

Founded by LeCompte, positivism has its roots in sociology and is used in most natural science studies. Researchers who employ positivism use the deductive approach where a hypothesis is tested. The positivists believe that knowledge is objective, the study environment should be controlled, and behaviour can be predicted and verified. Positivist studies focus on cause and effect relationships. Positivists are criticized for their lack of focus on meaning attributed to experiences, and also for not highlighting the social contexts of phenomena studied (Creswell, 1998; Patton, 2002; Polit & Hungler, 1995).

The critical paradigm was derived from interpretivism and seeks to answer research questions with an emphasis on 'change' or 'improve', and operates to reconstruct or deconstruct the social context through a participatory approach. Studies that align with the critical paradigm investigate sources and aspects of inequality in systems explored. Thus, the researcher is seen as an 'intellectual advocate' (LeCompte & Schensul, 1999 p. 45). Interpretivists and constructivists concede that the human mind and behaviour are independent of each other and cannot perfectly describe the reality of human consciousness and experiences (Schwandt, 1997).

The qualitative paradigm holds strongly to the examination and analysis of subjective experience of individuals and their constructions of the social world (Creswell, 1998; O'Reilly, 2005). Many other worldviews of qualitative research have been propounded. For example, the interpretivist/constructionist directs research activities to understand individual human action/behaviour with a focus on subjective meanings and interpretations. Thus, the interpretivists conclude that knowledge is constructed within the social domain and reality is ultimately subjective (O'Reilly, 2005; Saks & Allsop, 2007). Literature has identified other perspectives which emanate from the positivism and interpretivism that drive social research (Guba & Lincoln, 1994; LeCompte & Schensul, 1999).

This chapter focuses on the qualitative research approach because this approach is becoming popular of late among researchers at the University of Ghana. Also, over the years, faculty and graduate students of the School of Nursing, University of Ghana, have conducted research with a more qualitative orientation. For example, at this School, qualitative techniques have been employed to understand patients' experiences with mastectomy, hypertension, diabetes, infertility, and stroke, among others. The qualitative approach has also provided in-depth knowledge of health professional issues such as nurse-patient interaction, health professionals' attitudes towards post-operative pain management, and management of labour. The authors observe that the heavy qualitative orientation presupposes that nursing faculty should develop skills in quantitative research to afford better supervision of students interested in quantitative research. Also, nurse academics should be actively involved in multidisciplinary collaborative research where they can effectively contribute their qualitative expertise in such studies to fully understand the phenomenon under study.

Qualitative Research Approach

Nurse researchers using the qualitative approach choose from a variety of methodologies. The three foundational approaches employed in nursing research are phenomenology, ethnography, and grounded theory. The three approaches answer different research questions and they originated from different disciplines. This accounts for their distinct methodological foundations and perspectives. Other research approaches employed by nurse researchers include narrative enquiry, generic qualitative research, case studies, participatory action research, and community-based research. The nurse researcher should be open to different approaches as appropriate for a particular study (de Vos, Strydom, Fouché, & Delport, 2011; Caelli, Ray, & Mill, 2003; Creswell, 1998; Patton, 2002). Overviews of the three foundational qualitative approaches employed by nurse researchers are highlighted below.

Phenomenology: Phenomenology is derived from the Greek word 'phainomenon' which means 'appearing or to show self'. Husserl, a German philosopher, is identified as the proponent of this qualitative approach which originated from philosophy and is aimed at exploring lived experiences. Phenomenology is recognized as a philosophy and in the context of this paper, it is described as a research approach. The branches of phenomenology are Husserlian Transcendental Phenomenology and Heideggarian Hermeneutic Phenomenology. Husserlian phenomenology highlights bracketing, which requires the researcher to set aside prejudices, preconceptions, and beliefs to ensure that the phenomenon described is not influenced by the researcher's own ideas and beliefs. Heideggarian hermeneutics, however, embraces the personal interpretations of the researcher to understand and describe the lived experience under study. The main data collection method is in-depth interviews with open-ended questions. This enables participants to talk freely about their lived experience as in ways that enable the researcher to understand, describe, and interpret the participants' experience (de Vos et al., 2011; Creswell, 1998; Patton, 2002).

Grounded theory: The root of grounded theory is sociology and is aimed at generating a theory through systematic data collection and analysis. Theory generated through the application of grounded theory goes through a systematic process that is clarified in the research report and there is a link to the data generated through detailed descriptions. This approach was developed by Glaser and Strauss and is characterised by concurrent data analysis, theoretical sampling, emphasis on emerging theories and hypothesis, and recommended for studies where much is unknown. Grounded theory emphasises systematic data collection and analysis and does not accommodate insights gained from previous work. Also, grounded theory is associated with symbolic interaction which considers meaning and interpretation as important human processes. The nurse researcher employing a grounded theory approach leans on symbolic interaction for theory development (de Vos et al., 2011; Creswell, 1998; Patton, 2002).

Ethnography: Ethnography originated from anthropology and it was coined from two words 'ethno' which denotes folk and 'graph' derived from writing. Therefore, it refers to social scientific writing about particular folks or cultural groups. The methodology commenced with the research of Malinowski (1922) when he studied the social life of the Trobriand Islanders in the Western Pacific. Over the years, ethnographical studies have focused on tribes, subcultures, public and private organizations, and social problems. Ethnography seeks to understand a phenomenon being studied from the perspectives of the participant in the particular situation. This method emphasizes that a particular phenomenon is understood better in the local context due to the effect of the activities of particular individuals in a defined setting. It is also characterized by a fluid and flexible design. The researcher needs an extensive amount of field work to be able to understand the beliefs, views, and perspectives of the people being studied (O'Reilly, 2005; Silverman, 2001). Ethnography is considered the oldest qualitative methodology. However, the use of ethnographic methodology is relatively new in nursing and it is recorded that nurses

Chapter Twelve

started employing the methodology in the 1960s to learn and have a holistic contextual understanding of nursing phenomena (Buller & Butterworth, 2001; Oliffe, 2005; Roper & Shapira, 2000).

In a review, Roberts (2009) identified types of ethnography. In classical ethnography, for example, which is mainly used by anthropologists, the researcher has prolonged contact with the participants. In interpretive ethnography, the researcher tries to discover the meanings of social interaction; and in descriptive ethnography, the ethnographer describes what is happening. A focused ethnography may also be related to a time-limited exploration of a specific phenomenon (Muecke, 1994). Other authors refer to focused ethnography as mini-ethnography which is described as an ethnographic study with a specific focus. Other authors also identify autoethnography as a type of ethnography that has several terminologies enumerated by Patton, (2002, p.85), which involves investigating the researchers' own culture and recognizing the 'self' as an integral part of that culture and the complex nature of the culture is reported and discussed in relation to the self (Patton, 2002).

Leininger derived the ethnonursing methodology from ethnography and made a major contribution in the provision of appropriate transcultural nursing care. She asserted that different cultures perceive, know, and practice care in different ways; however, there are some commonalities about care among all cultures of the world. Leininger (1985) states that '*Ethnonursing has been conceptualized, developed and used as a specific research method focused primarily on documenting, describing, and explaining nursing phenomena*' (p. 38).

Sampling in Qualitative Research

Qualitative nurse researchers employ purposive, convenience, snowball, and theoretical sampling techniques as necessary. In purposive sampling, the researcher ensures that the participant that he/she believes has the desired experience is recruited. Convenience sampling involves sampling participants available during the time of recruitment and this type of sampling is sometimes referred to as accidental sampling. In snowball sampling, the researcher is led to other participants who meet the study criteria by those previously sampled, especially when the study involves, for example, groups with secret membership. Theoretical sampling is employed by grounded theorists to specifically sample appropriate informants during the process of data collection to fully develop an emerged theme or theory (Atkinson & Hammersley, 1998; O'Reilly, 2005; Silverman, 2001).

The sample size in qualitative studies is not large; recruitment stops when saturation (no new or little information is emerging from data) occurs and categories and themes are fully developed, especially in the case of grounded theory research. The aim of qualitative research is not to present what is representative of the wider population of interest but to have in-depth understanding of the phenomenon under study. Very large samples in qualitative studies do not guarantee depth of exploration.

Recruitment of study participants involves actual processes of involving participants who meet the inclusion criteria. It is noted that access to a field does not guarantee successful recruitment of participants as an individual may refuse to participate in a study even though the authorities or administrative leaders have granted approval for the study. Again, some social researchers give some form of incentive to aid the recruitment process in cases where it is difficult to recruit an adequate number of participants. This has been criticized for appearing to imply that such participants become part of the study because of the incentive and may provide wrong information to meet the inclusion criteria. These incentive-driven participants may give socially desirable information that could increase bias in the study results (Hammersley & Atkinson, 1995; O'Reilly, 2005).

Qualitative Methods of Data Collection

Qualitative research principles allow the researcher to use methods of data collection such as individual interviews, focus group discussion, observation, documentary and artefact review, and use of questionnaires. The data collection methods used in a particular study depends on the study objectives and the phenomenon under study. These data collection methods have been extensively examined in the literature and an overview of individual interviews is provided because it is considered the most common data collection methodologies in qualitative method (de Vos, et al., 2011; Patton, 2002; Roper & Shapira, 2000; Silverman, 2004; Spradley, 1979a, 1979b).

Individual interviews may be formal (planned and use of interview guide) or informal (unplanned interaction with participant); and these formal or informal interview may occur at scheduled times or be unscheduled according to the situation in the field. Interviews may be structured, semi-structured and unstructured depending on the type of research. Previous authors have dealt extensively with the types of questions asked during interviews such as descriptive, structural, and contrast questions (de Vos et al., 2011; Spradley, 1979a). Before interview sections, the researcher can have informal interactions with participants to enable them to relax before each formal planned interview session. Participants' background information can be obtained before interviews to provide further context and illumination to the findings. This also ensures that participants recruited meet the inclusion criteria, and that the range of participants required for the study objectives were recruited and interviewed (de Vos et al., 2011).

Semi-structured interviews also allow follow-up questions on participants' comments. Open-ended questions during qualitative interviews stimulate elaborate accounts from the participants. Strategic silence allows participants to reflect on their thoughts or questions asked during the interview. A conscious effort should be made to avoid leading questions that would produce any bias in the results. Interviews can last between 45 minutes and 90 minutes. The researcher should listen carefully and actively to participants' comments and restate or summarize participants' contributions during and at the end of interviews for confirmation that their views have been accurately captured. Non-verbal communications that might be a sign of discomfort or distress during interviews should be observed and appropriate interventions made. During the process of concurrent analysis, specific follow-up questions should be asked to help in the full development of emerging themes. The place and time of each interview should be at the convenience of the participant (Graneheim & Lundman, 2004; Hammersley & Atkinson, 1995; LeCompte & Schensul, 1999).

Qualitative Data Analysis (Practical Processes)

The literature gives general guidelines and processes for the management of qualitative data in a way that ensures rigour. Qualitative analysis requires investment of time and energy to make sense of the complex, voluminous data generated. The data generated in some qualitative studies are initially fragmented into smaller units to enable the researcher to categorise and make linkages between these smaller units (Graneheim & Lundman, 2004; Hammersley & Atkinson, 1995; Miles & Hubermann, 1994; Patton, 1990; Roper & Shapira, 2000; Strauss & Corbin, 1998). Individual approaches of qualitative research (phenomenology, ethnography and grounded theory) have specific steps for analysing generated data as indicated by previous researchers (Miles & Hubermann, 1994; Strauss & Corbin, 1998). This chapter focuses on general practical processes in qualitative analysis.

The transcripts are read several times along with personal reflections and field notes. Hence, data analysis occurs concurrently during the data collection to enable a follow-up on themes that emerge in the data. Identification of themes is done by reading through field notes, transcripts, and personal reflections several times to become immersed in the data and understand the participants' world (Krueger, 1998; Rabiee, 2004). Development of themes is done by seeking further explanations and dimensions of themes in the data generated through personal reflections. As this process continues, further data are collected from participants to answer or explain components of a theme where there is inadequate data.

Steps for qualitative data analysis are explicitly outlined by Burnard (1991) for thematic content analysis using manual processes. Notes taken during analysis include unique words, the context of the comments, the frequency of particular comments, whether comments are extensive, and how participants' comments are consistent or influenced by other participants (Krueger, 1998; Rabiee, 2004). It is noted that software for qualitative data management such as NVivo helps the researcher to manage data without following the processes of 'cut and paste'. The qualitative researcher employing qualitative software should remember that the software does not do the thinking for the researcher but only helps in handling voluminous data (LeCompte & Schensul, 1999).

After reading the transcripts, codes are assigned to segments of the text and the initial codes should be similar to terms used in the text. Similar codes are then grouped as the analysis progresses. During the process, there is sifting of data where data are separated into tree nodes and free nodes (when using the NVivo software). The free nodes involve data that are not directly related to the objectives of the study and the tree nodes comprise data related to the study objectives (Aziato, 2012). Similar patterns and variations among the groups are identified (Burnard, 1991; Morse & Field, 1996). As the analysis progresses, minor categories are grouped and later incorporated into major themes by re-grouping and collapsing similar minor themes (Burnard, 1991). The process of analysis is guided by the research questions, researcher reflections and discussions with research supervisor or experts in the field studied. The initial descriptive terms assigned to themes are changed to more abstract terms within the context of the relevant literature (Morse, 1994) to provide a link to the existing literature. After much sifting of data, the frameworks of main themes and sub-themes are developed and described. Morse (1994) considers thematic content analysis to involve four stages ,namely comprehending, synthesizing, theorizing, and recontextualizing. Nursing research also involves quantitative approaches and some highlights follow below.

Highlights of the Quantitative Research Approach and Methodology in Nursing

There are several quantitative research approaches that try to answer specific questions about nursing and health care in general. The quantitative approach is one in which the investigator primarily uses post-positivist claims for developing knowledge; that is, cause and effect thinking, reduction to specific variables and hypotheses and questions, use of measurement and observation, and the test of theories (Creswell, 2003). Quantitative research is mainly about populations and very essential in addressing selected questions associated with nursing such as effectiveness of nursing intervention. Thus, quantitative nursing research for example, tries to find out in this case the extent to which an intervention works. After the outcome of a particular medication has been verified on a number of the main population, this may provide reliable and objective results applicable to the larger population (de Vos et al., 2011).

It should be emphasized that the benefits of quantitative nursing research are observed in evidenced-based nursing care that seeks to employ scientific methods to find out interventions that are appropriate for the management of certain disease conditions. At the centre of evidence-based quantitative nursing research is the systematic and meaningful review of randomized research controlled trials. Quantitative research on nursing issues can utilize and build on previous research studies and gather a rich body of evidence about the extent to which effectiveness of different kinds of treatment can be measured (Patton, 1990). Quantitative nursing research also employs experimental studies with different design approaches such as the pre-test and post-test studies discussed by previous authors. In this way, the focus of nursing will be geared toward identification of factors responsible for both pre-test and post-test outcomes (Creswell, 2003).

Quantitative nursing research can also employ an observational approach where data are collected about the research participant but there is no chance or attempt by the researcher to alter the situation for any of the respondents and there is no associated intervention. Such an approach to quantitative research tries to describe and explain the magnitude of a disease, possibly including socio-demographic and clinical features of the people involved in the study who have that particular problem. It can also examine the relationship between features of participants and the level of their health, whether good or poor, which nursing can influence through health education. Quantitative cross-sectional study under the observational approach provides a snapshot in time as it is undertaken at a particular point in time but there is no follow up with the respondents (de Vos et al., 2011; Creswell, 2003). Nursing studies, for instance, can be carried out to find out about the prevalence of infection of a particular microorganism in a healthcare setting.

Nursing research could be designed in the form of cohort or longitudinal studies in which patients can be followed up over a period of time to find out what happens to them following treatment or other interventions. This type of quantitative nursing research looks at the causative agents and focuses on certain questions relating to phenomena A, B, C, and D. Specific questions could be whether C causes D, or how does C cause D, or does A influence B, or in what way does A relate to B or C? In this way, the nurse researcher will be able to identify specific links between causative agents and diseases. For example, this type of research may be able to identify the link between the development of cardiovascular diseases and individuals' smoking pattern (Parahoo, 2006).

In case control studies, participants are selected based on what has happened rather than what could happen, as in cohort or longitudinal studies. The cases are selected because they have the disease of interest to the nurse researcher. The control group, which is usually without the disease, is selected and related to socio-demographic variables such as sex, age, religion, marital status, occupation and type of accommodation. In such research, cases and controls are examined about their exposure to a particular causative factor and in each situation the causative factor(s) are compared (de Vos et al., 2011; Patton, 1990).

Quantitative research employs various sampling techniques described by previous authors, including random and non-random sampling techniques that best suit a particular research study. This approach rests on large sample sizes that enable generalization of findings. Nurses use special quantitative analysis packages to draw meaning and inferences from the data. The types of design and research questions inform the choice of appropriate statistical analysis to employ (Morse & Field, 1996; Parahoo, 2006; Patton, 1990).

Issues of Validity and Reliability/Rigour

The validity and reliability of a study is ensured by applying the key methodological principles. Reliability denotes the '*stability of research results and their ability to be replicated*' and validity involves '*whether or not researchers have actually discovered what they claim to have found, and the extent to which what they have learned can be applied to other populations*'

(Schensul, Schensul, & LeCompte, 1999, p. 271). In quantitative studies, validity and reliability are ensured through widely accepted standards and they have distinct procedures and principles that are applied through statistical analysis. However, validity and reliability issues have been debated in the literature where discourses involve the use of different criteria to establish the validity and reliability of qualitative research. This is based on the view that qualitative and quantitative studies operate from different worldviews; that the tenets of qualitative studies do not lend themselves to the use of specified principles and procedures for evaluation; and that the same criteria should be used to judge the validity and reliability of quantitative and qualitative studies (Hammersley, 1992; LeCompte & Schensul, 1999; Parahoo, 2006; Patton, 2002).

Perhaps the debate about the maintenance of validity and reliability in qualitative and quantitative researchers emanates from the language or terminologies used by the two paradigms. For example, qualitative researchers use rigour or trustworthiness - in contrast to the use of validity and reliability in quantitative studies - to denote why the findings of a particular study should be believed. Also, generalizability or external validity is used in quantitative research while transferability or fittingness is used in qualitative research to represent the applicability of findings in another similar context. The criterion of transferability in qualitative research has been debated to a large extent and there seems to be a concession that qualitative studies involve individual perceptions and the perception of the same individual may change over time. Therefore, different individuals in similar contexts may have different perceptions. Thus, transferability as a measure of rigour continues to be debated among social researchers (Cho & Trent, 2006; Mackenzie, 1994; Patton, 2002; Whittemore, Chase, & Mandle, 2001).

Qualitative researchers over the years have debated issues of validity and reliability because the principles and practice of qualitative research do not lend themselves to the positivists' emphasis on control that is used to describe principles of validity and reliability. It is recognized that the subjective perspective of the researcher during qualitative data collection and analysis and the naturalistic nature of data collection superimpose the 'control' in experimental studies. Therefore, the implementation of standard principles of validity and reliability becomes problematic (LeCompte & Schensul, 1999; Parahoo, 2006; Patton, 1999). The authors are of the opinion that all studies must ensure that the study is carried out with the necessary rigour to be valid and reliable. The nurse researcher should endeavour to adopt the appropriate techniques based on the type of study to ensure that findings that emanate from the study can be appreciated within a particular paradigm. Hence, Patton (1999) indicated that credibility of qualitative research depends on rigorous techniques and methods during collection and analysis, the credibility of the researcher based on training and experience, and the philosophical belief in the value of enquiry. Thus, studies that fail to observe rigour result in several such research cannot be trusted and the understanding of the phenomenon becomes blurred (Cho & Trent, 2006).

Strategies that are employed to achieve rigour in a particular study depend on the design of the study and the applicability of the strategy. Thus, researchers should be circumspect in their choice of strategies to ensure rigour. The key principles of rigour in qualitative studies such as credibility (whether results can be believed), transferability (compare results to similar context), dependability (repeatable or obtain similar results), and confirmability (results confirmed or corroborated by others) (Guba, 1981) are applicable in qualitative studies (de Vos et al., 2011; Atkinson & Hammersley, 1994; Polit & Hungler, 1999). Some of the measures employed by qualitative researchers to ensure rigour include: multiple data collection methods which allow triangulation, pilot study, memberchecks, maintaining an audit trail, ensuring prolonged fieldwork, using participant language, and employing an independent coder during data analysis as applied in a qualitative nursing research on pain management in Ghana (Aziato, 2012).

Ethical Considerations in Nursing Research

The nurse researcher employing either a quantitative or a qualitative approach is obliged to maintain high ethical standards during a particular study. Thus, research proposals are reviewed by credible boards and committees to ensure that the study is carried out within the appropriate ethical standards. We concede that even though the committee review is important, the researcher has the responsibility to ensure that the appropriate ethical standards are maintained during the study (LeCompte & Schensul, 1999; Murphy & Dingwall, 2001). Permission is sought from the institutions involved in the study according to administrative approval. Individual informed consent is sought from the individual participants by either signing or thumb-printing the consent form after the information has been fully explained in the language the participant understands.

Anonymity is ensured by assigning identification (ID) codes to all participants. Names mentioned or descriptions that could easily be identified in the research report are omitted to ensure privacy. Information shared by participants should be kept confidential and only those directly involved in the study (such as a transcriber, research assistant, and research supervisor or co-researchers) should have access to the raw data as necessary. The research data storing equipment such as a pen drive with interview files are kept under lock and key for a number of years consistent with ethical review board or institutional policies; for example, three-to-five years in case of any queries about the study. The storage equipment is destroyed according to laid down procedures. The hard copies of transcripts or questionnaires are also kept locked in a separate cabinet from the signed or thumb-printed consent forms so that information cannot easily be linked to a particular participant. The transcripts or questionnaires are anonymized by the use of ID codes. Computers used during the research should be password protected and files of raw data are password protected. The research assistants, transcribers or analysts involved in the study should complete a confidentiality agreement form to ensure commitment to maintaining confidentiality. Also, participants should be protected from harm during the study (Hammersley & Atkinson, 1995).

Critique of the Quantitative and Qualitative Research Approaches

Quantitative research is criticised for the following reasons: its inability to explain human experience; its insistence that the social environment always be controlled; the fact that the subjective nature of human experience cannot be 'measured'; the point also that human behaviour cannot always be predicted; and belief that the cause-effect relationship may be determined in all circumstances (Patton, 2002). The qualitative research approach has been criticised with regard to its unstructured design; subjectiveness; lack of rigour; and inability to provide generalizable findings. However, it is also contended that the core emphasis for qualitative studies is on what is happening rather than what is predicted (Creswell, 1998; LeCompte & Schensul, 1999a; Polit & Hungler, 1995).

Conclusion

Although many nurse researchers in Ghana and elsewhere advocate qualitative research, the authors emphasize that one should be guided by the research question and choose the appropriate research approach. This chapter aimed at providing practical processes of nursing research and the qualitative approach was given more attention because of the popularity of the approach among nurse researchers in Ghana. Indeed, most faculty members at the School of Nursing have conducted one study or another employing qualitative research approaches. The authors emphasize that nursing research has an enviable place in the field of both quantitative and qualitative research and rigorous processes should be employed to ensure valid and reliable outcomes. Such outcomes should be disseminated and published to enhance the development of nursing knowledge locally and internationally.

The authors are of the view that nurse researchers such as on the University of Ghana faculty, should be more proactive in conducting relevant, high-impact research that would enhance the visibility of nurses as researchers. The need for collaborating with other disciplines for related health research cannot be overemphasized. Thus, nurses who form the bedrock of healthcare and have access to patients and their families should take the challenge and move nursing research forward. It is also necessary to involve nurse clinicians in conducting and disseminating research to enhance application of research findings. The authors recommend that nurse researchers should at all times be mindful that robust research and effective dissemination is the key to evidence-based practice that aims to enhance patient and family care.

References

Algase, D.I & Whall, A.F. (1993). Rosemary Ellis' views on substantive structure of Nursing. *Image J Nurs Sch.* 1993 Spring; 25(1):69-72.

Atkinson, P., & Hammersley, M. (1998). Ethnography and Participant Observation. In N. K. Denzin & Y. S. Lincoln eds., *Strategies of Qualitative Inquiry* London: Sage. pp. 110-136.

Aziato, L. (2012). *Development of Clinical Guidelines for the Management of Post-Operative Pain within the Medico-Socio-Cultural Context of Ghana.* Bellville: University of the Western Cape.

Buller, S., & Butterworth, T. (2001). Skilled Nursing Practice: A Qualitative Study of the Elements of Nursing. *International Journal of Nursing Studies,* 38(4), 405-417.

Burnard, P. (1991). A Method of Analysing Interview Transcripts in Qualitative Research. *Nurse Education Today,* 11, 461-466.

Caelli, K., Ray, L. & Mill, J. (2003). Clear as Mud: Toward Greater Clarity in Generic Qualitative Research. *International Journal of Qualitative Methods,* 2(2).

Cho, J., & Trent, A. (2006). Validity in Qualitative Research Revisited. *Qualitative Research,* 6, 319-340.

Creswell, J.W. (2003). *Research Design: Qualitative, Quantitative and Mixed Methods Approaches.* Thousand Oaks: Sage.

Creswell, J. M. (1998). *Qualitative and Quantitative Inquiry and Research Design: Choosing Among Five Traditions.* Lodon: Sage.

Creswell, J. W. (1998). *Qualitative Inquiry and Research Design: Choosing Among Five Traditions.* London: Sage Publications.

de Vos, Strydom, H., Fouché, C. B., and Delport, C. S. L. (2011). *Research at Grass Roots: For the Social Sciences and Human Service Professions* 4th ed. Pretoria: Van Schaik Publishers.

Denzin, N. K., & Lincoln, Y. S. (1998). Entering the field of qualitative research.In: Denzin,N. K. and Lincoln,Y. S. eds. *Strategies of Qualitative Inquiry.* London: Sage, pp. 1-34.

Graneheim, U. H., & Lundman, B. (2004). Qualitative Content Analysis in Nursing Research: Concepts, Procedures and Measures to Achieve Trustworthiness. *Nurse Education Today,* 24(2), 105-112.

Guba, E. G., Lincoln, Y. S. (1994). Competing Paradigms in Qualitative Research. In N. K. Denzin and Y. S. Lincoln, eds. *The Lanscape of Qualitative Research: Theories and Issues*. Thousand Oaks: Sage, pp. 105-117.

Guba, L. (1981). Criteria for Assessing the Trustworthiness of Naturalistic Inquiries. *Educational Communication and Technology Journal, 29*, 75-92.

Hammersley, M. (1992). *What's Wrong with Ethnography: Methodological Explorations*. London: Routledge.

Hammersley, M., & Atkinson, P. (1995). *Ethnography: Principles in Practice*. 2nd ed. London: Routledge.

Heitkemper, M. M. (2007). The Past and Future of Nursing Research. *Asian Nursing Research, 1*(1), 4-10.

Krueger, R. (1998). *Analysing and Reporting Focus Group Results: Focus Group Kit 6*. London: Sage.

LeCompte, M. D., & Schensul, J. J. (1999). *Designing and Conducting Ethnographic Research: Ethnographer's Toolkit 1*. London: Altamira Press/Sage Publications.

Leininger, M. (1985). Ethnography and Ethno-nursing: Models and Modes of Qualitative Data Analysis. In Leininger, M. M. ed. *Qualitative Research Methods in Nursing*. New York: Grune and Stratton, pp. 33-71.

Mackenzie, A. E. (1994). Evaluating Ethnography: Considerations for Analysis. *Journal of Advanced Nursing, 19*(4), 774-781.

Miles, M. B., & Hubermann. (1994). *Qualitative Data Analysis: An Expanded Source Book*. 2nd ed. Newberg Park: Sage.

Morse, J. M. (1994). Emerging from the Data: The Cognitive Processes of Analysis in Qualitative Inquiry. In: Morse, J. M. ed. *Critical Issues in Qualitative Research Methods*. London: Sage, pp. 23-43.

Morse, J. M., & Field, P. (1996). *Nursing Research: The Application of Qualitative Approaches*. 2nd ed. London: Chapman and Hall.

Muecke, M. A. (1994). On the Evaluation of Ethnographies. In: Morse, J. M. ed. *Critical Issues in Qualitative Research Methods*. London: Sage, pp. 187-209.

Murphy, E., & Dingwall, R. (2001). The Ethics of Ethnography. In Atkinson, P., Coffey, A., Delamont, S., Lofland, J. and Lofland, L. eds. *Handbook of Ethnography*. London: Sage Publications. pp. 339-351.

Nelson, C., Treichler, P., & Grossberg, L. (1992). Cultural Studies. In: Grossberg, L., Nelson, C. & Treichler, P. eds. *Cultural Studies* (pp. 1-16). New York: Routledge.

O'Reilly, K. (2005). *Ethnographic Methods*. London: Routledge Taylor and Francis Group.

Oliffe, J. (2005). Demystifying Nursing Research. Why Not Ethnography? *Urologic Nursing, 25*(5), 395-399.

Parahoo, K. (2006). *Nursing Research: Principles, Process and Issues*. 2nd ed. Basingstoke: Palgrave Macmillan.

Patton, M. Q. (1990). *Qualitative Evaluation and Research Methods*. 2nd ed. Newbury Park, Sage.

Patton, M. Q. (2002). *Qualitative Research and Evaluation Methods*. London: Sage Publications Inc.

Polit, D. F., & Hungler, B. P. (1995). *Nursing Research: Principles and Methods*. 5th ed. Philadelphia: J.B. Lippincott Company.

Polit, D. F., & Hungler, B. P. (1999). *Nursing Research: Principles and Methods*. 3rd ed. Philadelphia: J.B. Lippincott Company.

Rabiee, F. (2004). Focus-group Interview and Data Analysis. *Proceedings of the Nutrition Society, 63*, 655-660.

Roberts, T. (2009). Understanding Ethnography. *British Journal of Midwifery, 17*(5), 291-294.

Roper, J. M., & Shapira, J. (2000). *Ethnography in Nursing Research*. Newberg Park: Sage Publications.

Saks, M., & Allsop, J. (2007). *Researching Health: Qualitative, Quantitative and Mixed Methods*. London: Sage.

Schensul, S. L., Schensul, J. J., and LeCompte, M. D. (1999). *Essential Ethnographic Methods: Observations, Interviews, and Questionnaires - Ethnographer's Toolkit 2*. London: Altamira Press/Sage Publications.

Schwandt, T. A. (1997). *Qualitative Inquiry: A Dictionary of Terms*. London: Sage.

Silverman, D. (2001). *Interpreting Qualitative Data: Methods for Analysing Talk, Text and Interaction*. 2nd ed. London: Sage.

Silverman, D. (Ed.). (2004). *Qualitative Research : Theory, Method and Practice* (2nd ed.). London: Sage.

Spradley, J. P. (1979). *The Ethnographic Interview*. Austin: Holt, Rinehart and Winston.

Strauss, A., & Corbin, J. (1998). Grounded Theory Methodology: An overview. In N. K.

Whittemore, R., Chase, S. K., & Mandle, C. L. (2001). Validity in Qualitative Research. *Qualitative Health Research, 11*, 522-537.

Index